# FOOT AND ANKLE PAIN

Other titles by Rene Cailliet from F. A. Davis Company:

**Hand Pain and Impairment, 4th Edition**
**Head and Face Pain Syndromes**
**Knee Pain and Disability, 3rd Edition**
**Low Back Pain Syndrome, 5th Edition**
**Neck and Arm Pain, 3rd Edition**
**Pain, Mechanisms and Management**
**Scoliosis: Diagnosis and Management**
**Shoulder Pain, 3rd Edition**
**Soft Tissue Pain and Disability, 3rd Edition**
**The Shoulder in Hemiplegia**
**Understanding Your Backache**

# FOOT AND ANKLE PAIN

## EDITION 3

### RENE CAILLIET M.D.

Professor Emeritus and Chairman
Department of Physical Medicine
 and Rehabilitation
University of Southern California
School of Medicine
Los Angeles, California

Illustrations by Rene Cailliet, M.D.

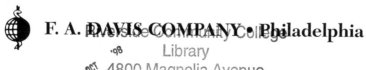

F. A. DAVIS COMPANY • Philadelphia

F. A. Davis Company
1915 Arch Street
Philadelphia, PA 19103

RD 781 .C33 1997

Cailliet, Rene.

Foot and ankle pain

.......................................................I. McKelvie
*Cover Designer*: Louis J. Forgione

As new scientific information becomes available through basic and clinical research, recommended treatments and drug therapies undergo changes. The author(s) and publisher have done everything possible to make this book accurate, up to date, and in
accord with accepted standards at the time of publication. The authors, editors, and publisher are not responsible for errors or omissions or for consequences from application of
the book, and make no warranty, expressed or implied, in regard to the contents of the
book. Any practice described in this book should be applied by the reader in accordance
with professional standards of care used in regard to the unique circumstances that may
apply in each situation. The reader is advised always to check product information (pack-
age inserts) for changes and new information regarding dose and contraindications
before administering any drug. Caution is especially urged when using new or infre-
quently ordered drugs.

**Library of Congress Cataloging in Publication Data**

Cailliet, Rene.
    Foot and ankle pain / Rene Cailliet. — Ed. 3.
        p.   cm.
    Includes bibliographical references and index.
    ISBN 0-8036-0216-2 (alk. paper)
    1. Foot—Abnormalities.   2. Foot—Diseases.   3. Foot—Wounds and
injuries.   4. Pain.   5. Ankle—Wounds and injuries.   I. Title.
    [DNLM: 1. Ankle Injuries.   2. Foot Diseases.   3. Foot Injuries.
WE 880 C134f 1997]
RD781.C33      1997
617.5′85—dc21
DNLM/DLC
for Library of Congress                                          96-46127

# Preface

As stated in the first volume of *Foot and Ankle Pain*, man's foot is subjected to daily stresses and strains. When impaired it lends itself to careful and meaningful examination as all the bones, ligaments, and muscles of the human foot are accessible to examination, palpation, and mechanical evaluation, unlike other extremity structures of the human body.

Much has been learned of foot function and malfunction since the first edition in 1983, thus prompting a new edition. In this volume the precise technique of manual examination will constitute a separate chapter to elucidate that premise.

Newer aspects of neurophysiology that apply to most neuromusculoskeletal components of the body will be applied to the foot and ankle, making its study more scientific and clinically meaningful.

Other clinical conditions, such as reflex sympathetic dystrophy and the latest diabetic conditions, will be highlighted.

Illustrations will be augmented in this volume, as their presence has been a major factor in the success of other volumes of the Cailliet Pain Series.

**RENE CAILLIET M.D.**

# Contents

# Illustrations

# CHAPTER 1

# Structural Functional Anatomy

The foot's 26 bones include 14 phalanges, 5 metatarsals, and 7 tarsal bones. The foot can be divided into three functional segments (Fig. 1–1). The posterior segment, which consists of the talus and calcaneus, is at the apex of the foot and is part of the ankle joint. It basically supports the body by its articulation on the tibia within the ankle mortise. The calcaneus is the posterior portion of the foot that is in direct contact with the ground.

The middle segment of the foot consists of the 5 tarsal bones, that is, the navicular, the cuboid, and 3 cuneiforms, which form an irregular rhomboid. The anterior segment contains 5 metatarsal bones and 14 phalangeal bones forming the toes. There are 2 phalangeal bones in the big toe and 3 in each of all others.

## THE ANKLE JOINT

The malleoli of the tibia and fibula form the mortise into which fits the talus, which functions as a hinge joint albeit at an angle as the mortise is laterally angled since the medial malleolus is anterior to the lateral malleolus in the transverse plane (Fig. 1–2).

In walking, the weight of the body is transmitted to the talus via the tibia. The fibular malleolus forms the lateral aspect of the ankle mortise but is not weight-bearing.

The foot articulates within the ankle mortise by virtue of contraction of the triceps surae (two heads of the gastrocnemius and soleus muscles), which causes *plantar flexion*, and the anterior crural muscles, which causes *dorsiflexion* (Fig. 1–3). The upper surface of the talus is convex and the undersurface of the tibia is concave, thus allowing rotational gliding at that articulation.

The body of the talus is wedged-shaped with the widest portion anterior. As the ankle dorsiflexes within the mortise, the wider portion comes up

1

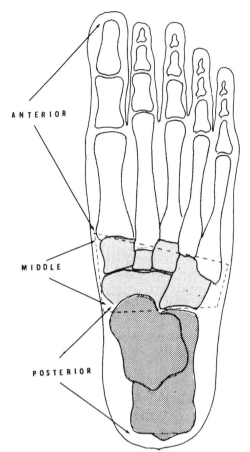

ANTERIOR

MIDDLE

POSTERIOR

**Figure 1–1.** The three functional segments of the foot.

between the two malleoli and wedges between them. Plantar flexion causes the smaller, posterior part of the talus to be within the mortise, allowing some lateral motion to occur. In the plantar position, the talus has movement that makes the joint "unstable," placing all of the support on the ligaments.

The ankle mortise is flexible as the tibia and fibula separate, and the fibula ascends when widened to physiologic limits by virtue of the oblique angle of the tibiofibular ligament (Fig. 1–3).

Dorsiflexion and plantar flexion of the ankle occur about an axis which passes through the body of the talus (Figs. 1–4 and 1–5). The line of the axis passes the tip of the fibula and is centrally located between the attachments of the lateral collateral ligaments (Fig. 1–6).

The ankle joint receives its strongest support from the collateral ligaments. The lateral collateral ligaments support the lateral aspect of the ankle, minimizing inversion. They are composed of three bands: (1) the anterior talofibular lig-

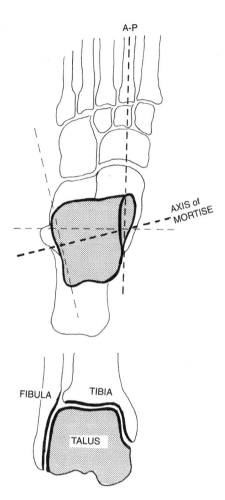

**Figure 1–2.** Superior view of the talus. Viewed from above, the talus is wedged-shaped, being wider anteriorly. It fits between the tibial and fibular malleoli, which form the ankle mortise.

ament, which originates from the neck of the talus and attaches to the tip of the fibula (Fig. 1–7); (2) the calcaneofibular ligament, which runs from the calcaneus to the tip of the fibula; and (3) the posterior talofibular ligament, which runs from the body of the talus to the tip of the fibula.

The anterior talofibular and calcaneofibular ligaments are the ligaments most frequently injured in ankle *inversion* sprains. This is because with the foot plantar-flexed, the talus is most unstable in the ankle mortise and thus most dependent on ligament support.

The medial aspect of the ankle joint is strongly supported by the medial collateral ligaments, termed the *deltoid* ligament. This ligament is composed of four bands: (1) the tibionavicular, (2) the anterior talotibial, (3) the calcaneotibial, and (4) the posterior talotibial ligament. These bands course from the medial malleolus to the navicular, the sustentaculum tali, and the posterior

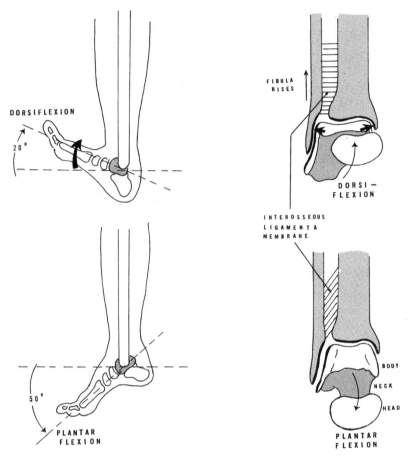

**Figure 1–3.** Motions of the talus within the mortise. The foot undergoes dorsiflexion and plantar flexion within the ankle mortise. As the foot dorsiflexes, the anterior, wider portion of the talus wedges into the mortise, widening the talofibular joint space and causing the talofibular ligament to become horizontal. This limits the degree of dorsiflexion. As the foot plantar flexes, the narrow posterior portion of the talus presents itself within the mortise and the talofibular joint narrows as the interosseous ligament resumes its normal oblique direction.

aspect of the talus. The deltoid ligament is strong and resists significant eversion injuries.

The axis of rotation, which was mentioned earlier (see Figs. 1–3 and 1–4), influences the stability of the collateral ligaments (see Fig. 1–5). Because the axis of rotation is at the tip of the fibula, it is central to all of the bands of the lateral collateral ligament, thus allowing them to remain taut during all motions. The medial end of the axis of rotation is eccentric to the point of attachment of all the medial

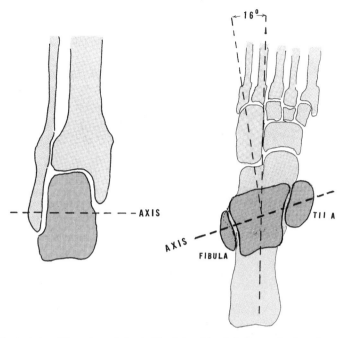

**Figure 1–4.** Axis of Rotation of the Ankle Joint. The left figure depicts the mortise of the ankle joint depicting the malleoli. The right figure shows the 16 degree angulation of the talus within the mortise.

bands of the deltoid ligament. The posterior medial ligament becomes taut on dorsiflexion, and the anterior medial ligament becomes taut on plantar flexion. This restricts the range of motion of dorsiflexion and plantar flexion, but the ligament does not sustain damage since the medial ligamentous bands are very strong.

## TALOCALCANEAL JOINT

Much of the inversion and eversion of the foot occurs at this joint. The entire body and part of the head of the talus rest on the anterior two thirds of the calcaneus, which is divided into three areas: (1) the posterior third, which is saddle-shaped; (2) the anterior third, which forms a horizontal surface; and (3) the intermediate third, which forms an inclined plane between the two other areas.

The talocalcaneal joint (subtalar) contains several joints in different planes, which permits simultaneous motion in different directions (Fig. 1–8). The posterior joint on the superior surface of the calcaneus is convex, and the joint surface on the inferior aspect of the talus is concave. This relationship allows inversion and eversion. Most of ankle inversion and eversion occurs within the taleocalcaneal joint as the talus is "locked" within the ankle mortise.

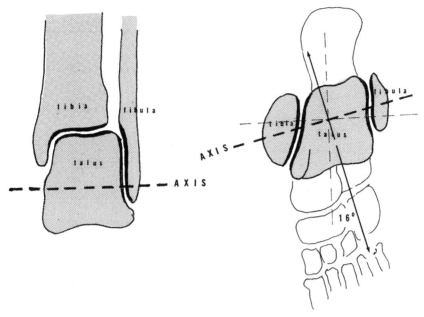

**Figure 1–5.** Ankle mortise and talar relationship. The axis of rotation about which the talus rotates within the ankle mortise is shown on the left, viewed anteriorly. The axis passes through the tip of the tibia. Viewed from above (right figure), the axis passes anteriorly to the fibula, forming an external "toe out" of 16°.

The entire body and part of the head of the talus rest on the anterior two thirds of the calcaneus and projects slightly in front of it (Fig. 1–9).

The anterior facets of the subtalar joint (see Fig. 1–8) consist of two similar facets on the superior aspect of the calcaneus and the inferior aspect of the body and neck of the talus. Those on the talus are convex and those on the calcaneus concave, the opposite of the posterior facets.

A deep groove, which is termed the *tarsal sinus* (see Fig. 1–8), separates the posterior facets from the middle facets. Within the sinus reside the *interosseous talocalcaneal* ligament, which is formed by two bands: (1) the interosseous band and (2) the lateral talocalcaneal band.

## TALOCALCANEAL LIGAMENTS

There are two major ligaments connecting the talus to the calcaneus:

1. The interosseous talocalcaneal ligament, which is relatively weak.
2. The lateral talocalcaneal ligament, which is a mere slip.

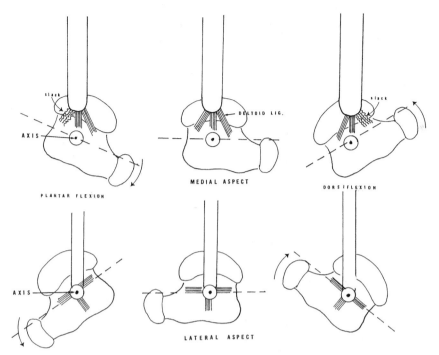

**Figure 1–6.** Relationship of medial and lateral collateral ligaments to the axis of rotation of ankle motion. The upper series of drawings shows the medial aspect of the ankle: the tibia upon the talus. The axis of rotation is eccentric to the tip of the tibia. As the ankle dorsiflexes, the anterior collateral ligaments become slack. Plantar flexion slackens the posterior collateral ligaments. The lower series of drawings shows the lateral aspect: the fibula to the talus. Because the axis of rotation is directly at the distal tip of the fibula, the collateral ligaments remain taut in all ankle motions.

Because these are weak ligaments, the talocalcaneal joint is more ably supported by the following:

3. The calcaneofibular portion of the lateral ligament of the ankle.
4. The calcaneotibial portion of the medial (deltoid) ligament of the ankle joint.

Support is also provided by the long tendons of the peroneus longus, peroneus brevis, flexor hallucis longus, tibialis posterior, and flexor digitorum longus.

All tendons crossing the ankle joint pass forward to insert on the foot: four tendons anterior to the joint axis and five behind.[1] These ligaments and joint surfaces resist forward displacement of the leg on the foot and ankle (Fig. 1–10).

The talocalcaneal joint is divided by the interosseous ligament into posterior and anterior portions. The posterior talocalcaneal joint has a synovial cavity

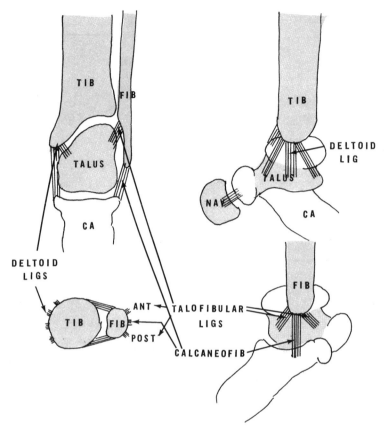

**Figure 1–7.** The collateral ligaments of the ankle joint. The ligaments of the ankle joint unite the tibia and the fibula (FIB) to the talus and calcaneus. The ligaments are termed according to the two or more bones to which they connect. NAV is the navicular bone. The upper left figure is the rear view; the right upper, the medial view; the left lower, the top view; and the right lower, the lateral view.

and is known as the *subtalar joint*. The anterior talocalcaneal joint shares a synovial cavity with the talonavicular joint, and hence is termed the *talocalcaneonavicular joint*.

This latter joint is formed superiorly by the posterior surface of the navicular; below by the middle and anterior facets of the talus; and between the navicular and the sustentaculum, by a firm ligament, the plantar calcaneonavicular ligament, termed the "spring" ligament (Fig. 1–11).

The interosseous talocalcaneal ligament runs the length of the tarsal tunnel, which, at its fibular end, thickens into a fibrous band that connects the two small tubercles opposing each other from the talus and the calcaneus. This firm band, termed the *ligamentum cervicis*, allows some rotation.

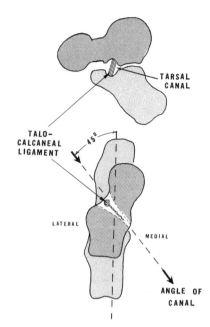

**Figure 1–8.** The subtalar (talocalcaneal) joint. The talus and the calcaneus are joined by three facets: the anterior, the middle, and the posterior. In its oblique course, the sinus tarsi (tarsal tunnel) contains the talocalcaneal ligament, which binds the two bones. The rounded end of the ligament is termed the cervicis ligament.

Because the interosseous talocalcaneal ligament runs perpendicular to the subtalar axis and the ligamentum cervicis lies laterally, it tenses during inversion of the foot and is slack during eversion. This increases the stability of the supinated foot, which is the objective of maintaining a stable foot. Clinically, when the foot is inverted, this ligament can be palpated at the large opening of the tarsal canal just anterior to the fibular malleolus.

Small bony processes (Fig. 1–12) located on the lateral inferior aspect of the body of the talus impinge on an opposing tubercle on the calcaneus, thus limiting inversion and eversion.

## TRANSVERSE TARSAL JOINT

The transverse tarsal joint consists of the talonavicular and the calcaneocuboid joints (Fig. 1–13). This joint, which has been termed the "surgeon's

**Figure 1–9.** Lateral aspect of talocalcaneal joint. The talus (T) is divided into the body (B), neck (N), and head (H). It articulates with the calcaneus (C). The tarsal sinus (TS) exists between them. The achilles tendon (AT) attaches to the posterior aspect of the calcaneus.

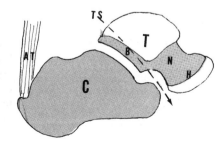

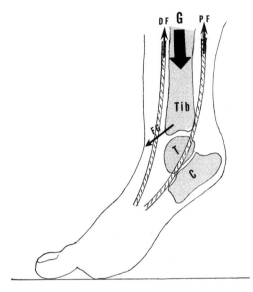

**Figure 1–10.** Prevention of anterior shear of leg on foot. The ligaments and muscles (dorsiflexors [DF] and plantar flexors [PF]) of the leg (tibia [Tib]) prevent anterior shear (forward glide [FG]), which is initiated by gravity (G) and downward rotation of the talus (T) upon the calcaneus (C). (Modified from Basmajian, JV: Grant's Method of Anatomy, ed. 8, The Williams & Wilkins Co., Baltimore, 1971, pp 406)

tarsal joint," the midtarsal joint, or Chopart's joint, is the frequent site of amputation of the foot.

Movements of the foot require definition as well as articular site:

*Supination and pronation* are rotations about the long (anteroposterior) axis of the foot.

*Adduction and abduction* are horizontal movements of the forepart of the foot away from the sagittal plane.

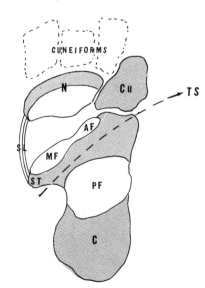

**Figure 1–11.** The bed for the talus on the calcaneus: The spring ligament (looking down on the calcaneus [C] with the talus removed). The navicular (N) shows the facet into which articulates the head of the talus. The middle facet (MF), anterior facet (AF), and posterior facet (PF) form the borders of the tarsal sinus (TS). The sustentaculum tali (ST) is the site of attachment of the spring ligament (SL). The cuboid (Cu) and the cuneiforms are shown for orientation.

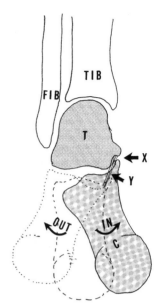

**Figure 1–12.** Motion of subtalar (talocalcaneal) joint. The talus (T) is fixed within the mortise of the tibia (TIB) and fibula (FIB). It articulates upon the calcaneus (C). Although limited, some lateral motion occurs at this joint. A bony process on the lateral inferior aspect of the body of the talus (X) impinges on the superior process of the calcaneus to limit inversion (IN). Eversion (OUT) is limited by a ligament between these two processes (Y).

*Inversion and eversion* are the turning of the sole to face the opposite sole. Inversion is a combination of supination and adduction, and eversion is a combination of pronation and abduction. Inversion and eversion are movements of the "entire foot" except the talus yet involve all the articulations below and in front of the talus and of the forepart of the foot on the hindpart.

## TALONAVICULAR JOINT

The rounded head of the talus fits into the cupped surface of the navicular. Motion is rotation about an axis through the talus, which slants in a forward, downward, and medial direction. Because the articular surface of the talus is wider than the articular surface of the navicular, it allows significant gliding at the talonavicular joint, allowing inversion and eversion. The two muscles of inversion (the tibialis anterior and posterior) and the three of eversion (peronei) insert in front of the transverse tarsal joint.

## CALCANEOCUBOID JOINT

These joints are accessory joints of inversion and eversion. The anterior surface of the calcaneus is rounded off (convex) medially, and the posterior surface of the cuboid is concave.

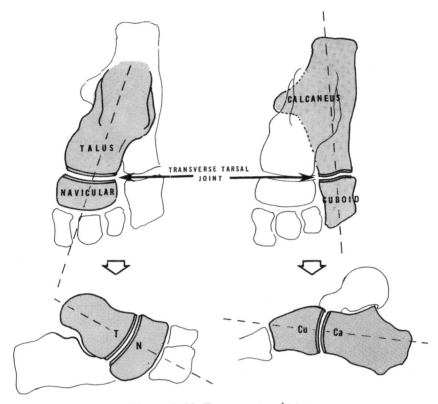

**Figure 1–13.** Transverse tarsal joint.

These joints are joined by two ligaments: the long plantar and the short plantar (Fig. 1–14). The long plantar ligament extends from the plantar surface of the calcaneus to the ridge of the cuboid. Its most superficial fibers extend further to attach to the bases of the second, third, fourth, and, occasionally, the fifth metatarsal. These fibers convert the groove of the cuboid into a tunnel that contains the peroneus longus tendon, which proceeds distally through a sulcus in the base of the fifth metatarsal bone.

The short plantar ligament extends from the anterior tubercle of the calcaneus to the cuboid. This ligament specifically unites the calcaneocuboid joint.

## THE ARCHES OF THE FOOT

The middle functional segment (see Fig. 1–1) consists of five tarsal bones: the navicular, the cuboid, and the three cuneiform bones. By their configuration and firm interosseous ligaments, they form a firm arch, with the middle

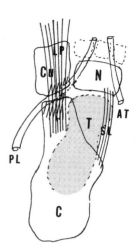

**Figure 1–14.** The three plantar ligaments. The long plantar ligament (LP) extends from the plantar surface of the calcaneus (C) to the cuboid (Cu), and its superficial fibers extend to the bases of the second, third, fourth, and fifth metatarsals (not shown). These fibers convert a groove in the cuboid into a tunnel for the peroneus longus tendon (PL). The short plantar ligament (not labelled) stretches from the anterior tubercle of the calcaneus to the cuboid. The spring ligament connects the calcaneus to the navicular.

cuneiform being the keystone (Fig. 1–15). These bones within the arch are "side-to-side" joints supported by ligaments (Fig. 1–16).

The *lateral longitudinal arch* (Fig. 1–17) is formed by the calcaneus, cuboid, and fourth and fifth metatarsals. It is a small arch, which bears the weight of stance in its early phase before the foot pronates to place weight upon the medial arch (see "Gait," Chap. 3). It can flatten at the hinge joint between the cuboid and the fourth and fifth metatarsals

The *medial longitudinal arch* is formed by the calcaneus, talus, navicular, three cuneiforms, and three medial metatarsals. It is a higher arch than the lateral, with its summit at the head of the talus and the navicular. The posterior tibialis tendon (Fig. 1–18), which inserts upon second, third, and fourth metatarsal bones at their base after passing under the spring ligament, may act as a sling for the arch. The medial arch may flatten at the "hinge" between the talus and the navicular bone.

The transverse arches of the foot (see Fig. 1–15) include the posterior metatarsal arch, which is created by the bases of the metatarsal bones and is also reasonably firm. The anterior metatarsal arch is flexible and flattens during phases of gait when weight bearing and during pronation and supination.

## JOINTS DISTAL TO THE TRANSVERSE JOINT

The anterior margin of the middle segment does not present a straight border articulating with the bases of the metatarsals. The second cuneiform is smaller and is thus set back, forming an indentation into which the base of the second metatarsal is wedged.

The second metatarsal bone being wedged between the first and third cuneiform can move only in a plantar flexion-extension direction. The bases of

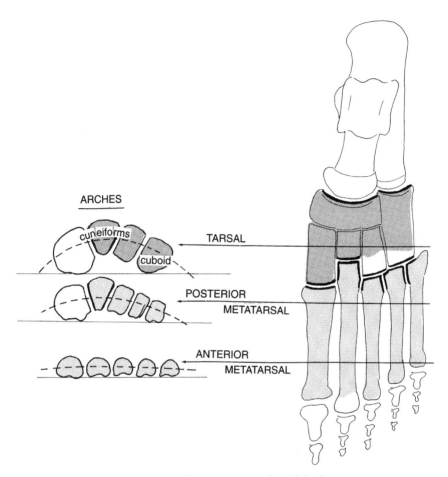

**Figure 1–15.** The transverse arches of the foot.

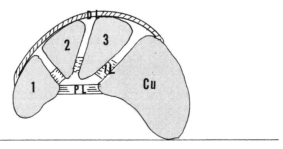

**Figure 1–16.** Side-to-side joint ligaments supporting the tarsal arch. The ligaments connect in a side-to-side manner the cuboid and the three cuneiforms.

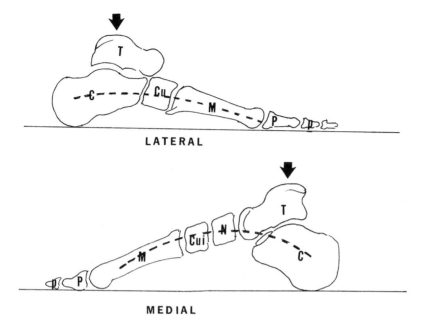

**LATERAL**

**MEDIAL**

**Figure 1–17.** The longitudinal arches. Viewed laterally, the longitudinal arch consists of the calcaneus (C), the cuboid (Cu), and the metatarsal (M). The phalanges (P and p) are not in the arch. The talus (T) bears the body weight (arrow). The medial longitudinal arch is formed by the calcaneus (C), talus (T), navicular (N), cuneiforms (Cui), and the three medial metatarsals (M).

the third, fourth, and fifth metatarsals are obliquely shaped, permitting rotatory motion of the third on the second, the fourth on the third, and the fifth on the fourth. The fifth metatarsal contacts only at the base of the fourth, and the cuboid proximally moves the greatest angulation. This allows "cupping" of the outer metatarsals, increasing their arch curvatures.

The first metatarsal is the thickest and shortest of the five metatarsal bones. It has a kidney-shaped base, which articulates on the distal area of the cuboid. This permits not only dorsal and plantar flexion but also rotation about the base of the second metatarsal bone and the first cuneiform. The anterior tibial and peroneus longus tendons attach to the plantar surface of the first metatarsal (Fig. 1–19).

Under the head of the first metatarsal are two small facets upon which articulate two small sesamoid bones. These sesamoid bones, erroneously called "accessory" bones, are incorporated within the tendons of the flexor hallucis brevis and act as fulcum in the function of the tendons. They also bear weight.

The forward projected length of the metatarsals follows a sequence of 2 > 3 > 1 > 4 > 5. The second metatarsal head normally protrudes the farthest, with the first metatarsal being shorter than the third (Fig. 1–20). Excessive

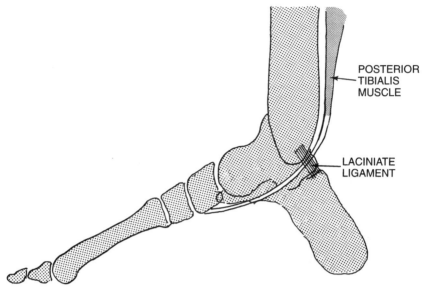

**Figure 1–18.** Posterior tibial tendon. The tibialis posterior muscle arises from the upper two thirds of the interosseous membrane and from the bones on each side of the membrane. Its tendon inclines medially to reach the fossa behind the medial malleolus, where it is covered by the laciniate ligament, forming a tunnel. This causes a pulley effect for the tendon, which attaches to the base of the second, third, and fourth metatarsal bones at their base. Its action is plantar flexion and inversion of the foot.

shortening of the first metatarsal, from whatever cause, may have pathologic significance since this causes the second metatarsal head to bear excessive weight during gait.

## METATARSOPHALANGEAL JOINTS

The phalanges articulate on the large convex articular surfaces of the metatarsal bones in a gliding manner (Fig. 1–21). The cartilaginous cover of the metatarsal heads extends from the plantar surface of the metatarsal heads onto the dorsum of the heads, allowing excessive dorsiflexion of the toes. In normal walking, the big toe "hyperextends" at every step, estimated to be 900 times in walking a mile.

There are two phalanges in the first (big) toe and three in all the others. For proper range of motion, the toes should be in a proper direct alignment with the capsules flexible and the tendons of appropriate length in their sheaths (Fig. 1–22).

The metatarsal bone projection—2 > 3 > 1 > 4 > 5—differs in the projection of the phalanges, which is normally 1 > 2 > 3 > 4 > 5 with the big toe projecting the farthest (see Fig. 1–20).

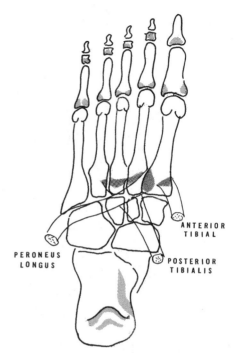

**Figure 1–19.** Tendon attachments on the first metatarsal bone. Viewed from the plantar surface, the anterior tibial tendon attaches to the medial aspect of the first metatarsal bone at its base. The peroneus longus tendon attaches to the lateral aspect of the first metatarsal. The posterior tibialis tendon attaches to the bases of the second, third, and fourth metatarsals.

PERONEUS
LONGUS

ANTERIOR
TIBIAL

POSTERIOR
TIBIALIS

The tendons act differently on the phalanges of the first toe as compared to those of the other four toes. Because the first toe has only two phalanges, the distal phalanx is caused to "press down" against the ground when flexed (Fig. 1–23). The other toes have three phalanges with the tendons crossing three joints, causing them to "grip" the ground surface.

## MUSCLES

Muscles that originate° away from the foot and act on the foot constitute the "extrinsic" foot muscles (Figs. 1–24 and 1–25), whereas the "intrinsic" foot muscles originate and insert within the foot itself (Figs. 1–26 through 1–29).

Of the major extrinsic muscles, the plantar flexors are the gastrocnemius and soleus muscles. The *gastrocnemius* originates above the knee by two

°The terms *origin* and *insertion* are used in most textbooks to describe muscular action with the distal appendage being free to move as the tendon and its muscle direct. This description varies with the specific muscle. For example, in the foot, when the foot is fixed to the floor, muscular action indicates that the leg muscles "originate" from the foot and "insert" into the lower leg. When the leg moves during the swing phase, the muscles "originate" from the leg and "insert" into the foot.

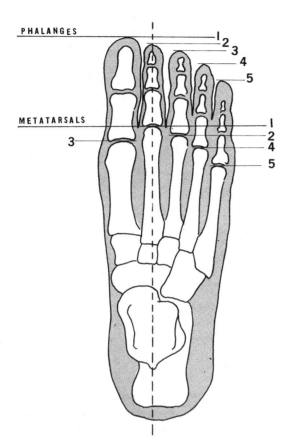

PHALANGES

METATARSALS

**Figure 1–20.** Relative length of projection of the metatarsals and the phalanges. The relative anterior protrusion of the metatarsals follows the pattern: 2 > 3 > 1 > 4 > 5. The second metatarsal is the longest and the first metatarsal the third longest. The phalangeal length patterns are l > 2 > 3 > 4 > 5, in which the first toe protrudes farther forward than the others that are in sequence.

heads with one connected to each femoral condyle. Halfway down the leg, the gastrocnemius ends in a flattened tendon, the *Achilles tendon,* which attaches to the posterior aspect of the calcaneus. With the foot weight bearing, the gastrocnemius-soleus muscle elevates the heel from the floor. With the leg elevated, it plantar flexes the foot on the lower leg. Because of the oblique angle of the ankle mortise (see Fig. 1–5), the gastrocnemius-soleus muscle is thus a powerful supinator of the subtalar joint when the foot is fixed on the floor.

The *soleus* muscle lies under the gastrocnemius and originates from the upper tibia and fibula below the knee joint. It also acts on the foot, but unlike the gastrocnemius, which is a two-joint muscle, the soleus does not have the ability to flex the knee. The soleus muscle ends within the deep portion of the Achilles tendon, midway down the leg.

With the foot fixed on the ground, the gastrocnemius-soleus group changes its origin and insertion relationship. The foot becomes the origin and

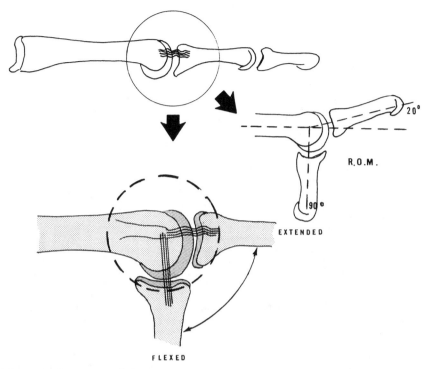

**Figure 1–21.** Metatarsal phalangeal joints. As a result of the eccentric radius of rotation about the axis of the head of the metatarsal (dashed circle), flexion of the phalanx is possible to greater than 90°. However, because there is cartilage on the superior aspect of the metatarsal head, hyperextension of the joint is possible.

the muscles move the tibia backward. With a flexed knee, the soleus becomes the prime ankle plantar flexor and the gastrocnemius becomes ineffective.

All the tendons that pass behind the malleoli are considered plantar flexors. Medially these are the tibialis posterior, flexor digitorum longus, and flexor

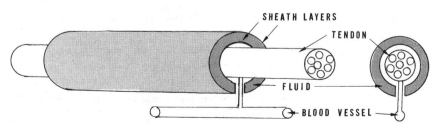

**Figure 1–22.** Tendon sheath (schematic). The tendon sheath has two layers—parietal and visceral—between which there is synovial fluid that acts as a lubricant. The blood supply to the tendon flows through a small blood vessel that enters through a fold in the sheath.

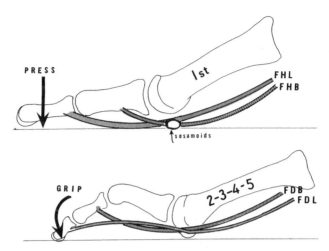

**Figure 1–23.** Action of the flexor tendons. The tendons of the big toe cross two joints and thus act by "pressing" the distal phalanx to the floor. The sesamoid bones are incorporated into the tendons of the flexor hallucis brevis (FHB) and act as a fulcrum for flexor action. The flexor tendons of the other toes cross three joints and act to "grip" the floor. This action is performed by the flexor digitorum brevis (FDB) and longus (FDL). FHL is the flexor hallucis longus.

hallucis longus. Laterally these muscles are the peroneus longus and brevis. These muscles exert merely 5% of the force needed to raise the heel from the floor. The gastrocnemius-soleus group is the primary mover.

As stated, the long digital flexors create the firm pressure of the toes on the ground. Furthermore, because the tendons run down the medial aspect of the ankle, they afford lateral stability of the ankle, minimizing eversion (Fig. 1–30).

If the body shifts laterally from the center of gravity (Fig. 1–31), the tendons on the medial side of the ankle pull the leg medially over the foot. These muscles are principally the *tibialis posterior* and *the tibialis anterior*.

The sensorimotor action that implements this "righting" action of the foot-ankle stance is the sensory feedback mechanism of the neuromuscular system (Fig. 1–32).

The extrinsic muscles acting on the foot and ankle are divided into three groups: lateral, anterior, and medial. The *lateral group* contains the peroneus longus and peroneus brevis, which arise from the lateral aspect of the fibula. The peroneus longus arises higher on the fibula and is the most superficial. Both muscle tendons share a common synovial sheath as they pass behind the lateral malleolus. The peroneus brevis attaches to the base of the fifth metatarsal, while the peroneus longus runs deeply across the plantar surface of the foot to attach to the base of the first metatarsal (see Fig. 1–19). Their primary function is to evert the ankle.

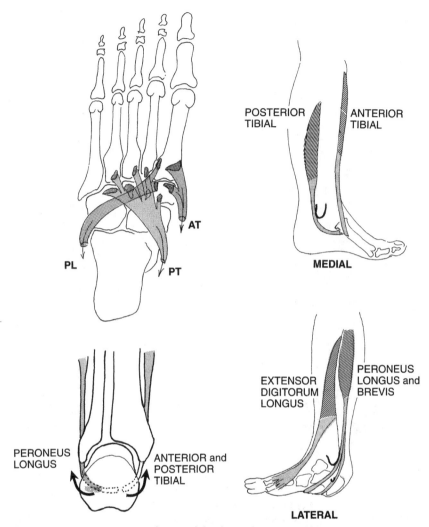

**Figure 1–24.** Extrinsic musculature of the foot. The origin, direction, and insertion of the extrinsic muscles acting upon the foot are shown. The anterior tibial (AT) and the posterior tibial (PT) are medial muscles that invert the foot. The peroneus longus (PL) everts the foot. Both the posterior tibial and the peroneus longus also plantar flex the foot. The extensor digitorum and the anterior tibial dorsiflex the foot.

The *anterior group* of extrinsic muscles comprises the extensor digitorum longus, peroneus tertius, extensor hallucis longus, and tibialis anterior. The *tibialis anterior* originates from the lateral aspect of the tibia and crosses the dorsum of the foot medially to insert on the medial cuneiform and the base of the first metatarsal. Its action is to invert and dorsiflex the foot on the ankle (Fig. 1–33).

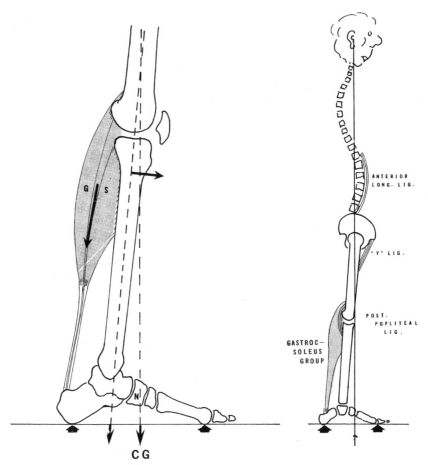

**Figure 1–25.** Muscular effort of relaxed two-legged standing position. In standing on both feet in a relaxed manner, the spine leans on the anterior longitudinal ligament, the hip on the iliofemoral (Y) ligament, and the knees extend to lean on the posterior popliteal ligaments. The gastrocnemius-soleus must maintain tonus to pull the leg back because the center of gravity falls some 3° ahead of the talus. Relaxed erect posture is principally ligamentous with only the gastrocnemius-soleus group active. (From Cailliet, R.: Low Back Pain Syndrome, ed. 3. F.A. Davis, 1968, with permission.)

The *extensor digitorum longus* arises from the entire length of the anterior surface of the fibula and from the interosseous membrane and deep fascia. It inserts into the distal two phalanges of the lateral four toes. The lower fourth of this unipennate muscle is known as the *peroneus tertius*, which attaches on the dorsum of the fourth and fifth metatarsals. It is an everter of the foot.

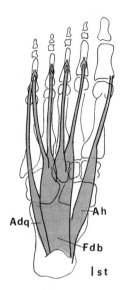

**Figure 1–26.** Intrinsic muscles of the sole of the foot: first layer. Adq = abductor digiti quinti; Ah = abductor hallucis; Fdb = flexor digitorum brevis.

The *extensor hallucis longus* arises from the middle two-thirds of the anterior surface of the fibula and the interosseous membrane. It inserts onto the base of the distal phalanx of the hallux.

The *extensor digitorum brevis* arises from the anterior upper surface of the calcaneus and the extensor retinaculum. The extensor retinaculum is divided into two segments (Fig. 1–34). The superior extends from the medial lower

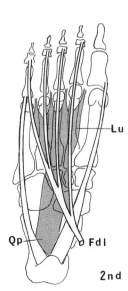

**Figure 1–27.** Intrinsic muscles of the sole of the foot: second layer. Qp = quadratus plantae; Lu = lumbricales; Fdl = flexor digitorum longus.

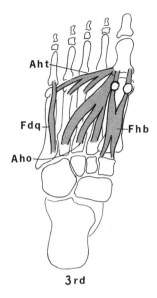

**3rd**

**Figure 1–28.** Muscles of the sole of the foot: third layer. Aht = Adductor hallucis: transverse head; Aho = Adductor hallucis: oblique head; Fhb = Flexor hallucis brevis; Fdq = Flexor digiti quinti brevis.

aspect of the fibula, attaches to the medial aspect of the lower tibia, and covers the anterior tibialis. The lower segment forms a Y-shaped band that contains the tendons of the peroneus tertius, extensor digitorum longus, and extensor hallucis longus. It prevents bowing of these tendons when they are contracted. The superior peroneal retinaculum attaches from the lateral distal malleolus and contains the peroneal tendons.

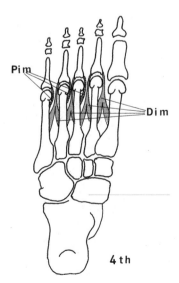

**4th**

**Figure 1–29.** Intrinsic muscles of the sole of the foot: fourth layer. Pim = plantar interosseous muscles; Dim = dorsal interosseous muscles.

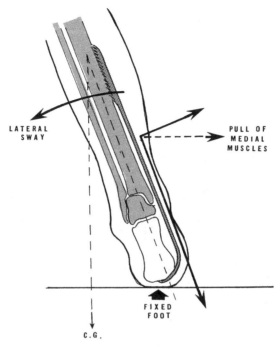

**Figure 1–30.** Muscular action giving lateral stability in one-legged stance. As the body moves laterally from the center of gravity (CG), the medial muscles (tibialis anterior and tibialis posterior) act to pull the body medially. Their action originates at the foot and inserts upon the leg (arrows).

## THE POSTERIOR GROUP

The posterior group of lower leg muscles is also termed the *posterior crural muscles* (Fig. 1–35). These muscles are divided into two groups: *superficial* and *deep*.

The superficial group includes the gastrocnemius, plantaris, and soleus. The gastrocnemius has two bellies covering the popliteal fossa. The soleus arises from the lower limits of the fossa, and the plantaris lies between them (Fig. 1–36). All three blend into an aponeurosis forming the Achilles tendon, which attaches to the posterior superior aspect of the os calcis (calcaneus), causing it to rise during gait. All three muscles are served by the tibial nerve.

A bursa lies between the semimembranosus muscle and the medial head of the gastrocnemius. This bursa communicates with a bursa between the gastrocnemius and the knee capsule. Injury (sprain) of the gastrocnemius muscle can cause effusion in the knee joint.

The plantaris muscle lying between the gastrocnemius and soleus muscles has a 1-foot-long tendon that arises near the lateral head of the gastrocnemius muscle and inserts on the medial aspect of the Achilles tendon.

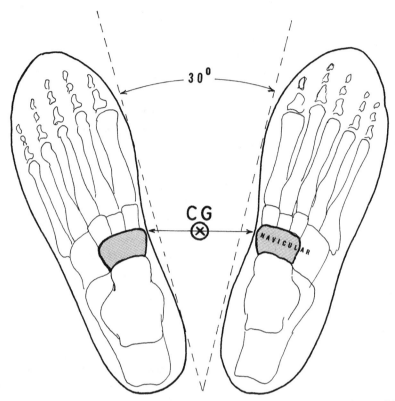

**Figure 1–31.** Center of gravity in two-legged stance. With the person standing and balancing on both feet, the feet describe an arc with the feet "toeing out" 30°. The center of gravity (CG) of the body is midway between the two navicular bones.

The *soleus* is so termed because it is shaped like the sole of a shoe. The soleus originates in a horseshoe-shaped line on the posterior aspect of the upper tibia. As a plantar flexor, it is more powerful than the gastrocnemius muscle.

As shown in Figure 1–31, the center of gravity passes 3° in front of the talus, and the gastrocnemius-soleus group pulls the leg back to maintain balance (Fig. 1–37). As the center of gravity of the body shifts forward, the posterior group of the lower leg muscles pulls the leg backward and the anterior group pulls the leg forward.

## THE DEEP MUSCLES

The *plantaris* muscle originates from a tendon on the lateral epicondyle of the femur and runs backward to insert on the posterior aspect of the tibia. It runs between the fibular (lateral) collateral ligament of the knee and the lateral meniscus (Fig. 1–38).

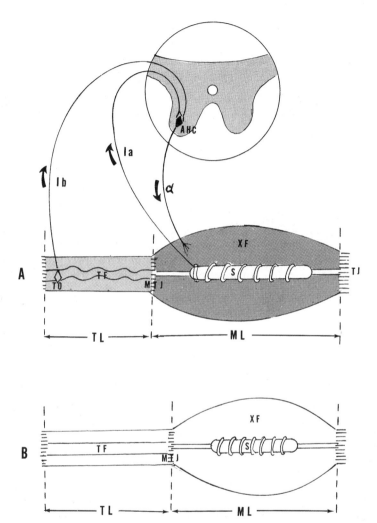

**Figure 1–32.** Musculotendinous mechanism. (A) The spindle system (S) measures the length of the muscle (ML), and the tendon organs (Golgi) (TO) monitor the tension. Stretching the spindle system activates the Ia fiber, whereas stretching the tendon organ activates the Ib fibers. These influence the anterior horn cells (AHC), which send motor fiber activity via the alpha fibers to the extrafusal fibers (XF). With the muscle at resting level (A), the tendon fibers (TF) are slightly coiled. When the extrafusal fibers contract (B), the muscle (ML) shortens, and the tendon elongates (TL) to the degree that the tendon fibers can elongate. The tendon fibrils (TF) composed of collagen fibers uncoil. Excessive muscle contraction can tear the muscle-tendon juncture (MTJ).

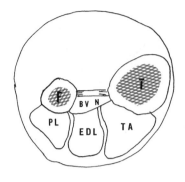 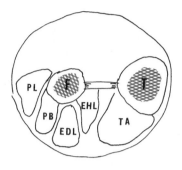

**UPPER THIRD**          **LOWER THIRD**

**Figure 1–33.** Sections through the lower leg: Anterior leg muscles. The *upper third* contains the tibialis anterior (TA), peroneus longus (PL), and extensor digitorum longus (EDL). The blood vessels (BV) and nerves (N) are contained in the compartment formed by muscle fascia. The *lower third* contains the tibialis anterior (TA); extensor hallucis longus (EHL); extensor digitorum longus (EDL), which contains the peroneus tertius (not shown); peroneus brevis (PB); and peroneus longus (PL). The tibia (T) and the fibula (F) form the lower leg.

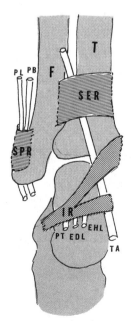

**Figure 1–34.** Extensor and peroneal retinaculum. The retinacula that are located in the front of the ankle (tibia [T], fibula [F]) are divided into the superior extensor retinaculum (SER); inferior retinaculum (IR), formed in a Y shape; and superior peroneal retinaculum (SPR). They contain the tendons that traverse the front of the ankle to keep the ankles from bowing.

TA   = tendon anterior
PL   = peroneus longus
PB   = peroneus brevis
PT   = peroneus tertius
EDL = extensor digitorum longus
EHL = extensor hallucis longus

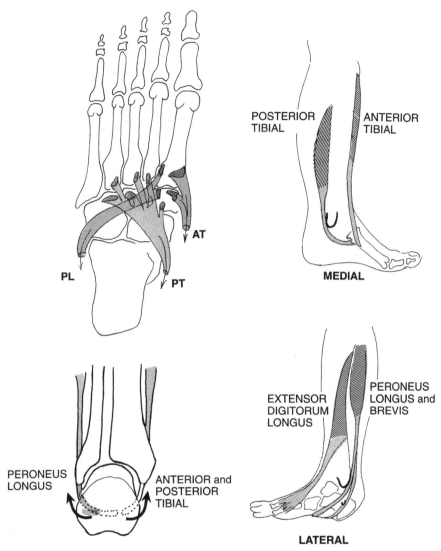

**Figure 1–35.** Extrinsic musculature of the foot. The origin, direction, and insertion of the extrinsic muscles acting upon the foot are shown. The anterior tibialis (AT) and posterior tibialis (PT) muscles are medial muscles that invert the foot. The peroneus longus (PL) everts the foot. Both the posterior tibial and peroneus longus also plantar-flex the foot. The extensor digitorum longus and the anterior tibialis muscles also dorsiflex the foot.

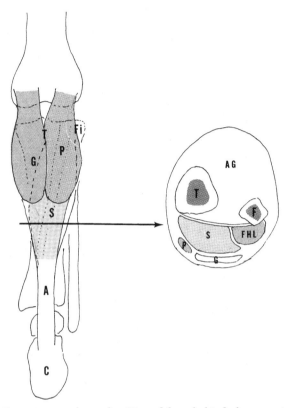

**Figure 1–36.** Posterior crural muscles. Viewed from behind, the posterior crural muscles are the gastrocnemius (G), soleus (S), and plantaris (P). A is the Achilles tendon; C, calcaneus; T, tibia; and Fi, the fibula. The long arrow divides the lower leg with the right-hand figure being a transverse section through the leg. G is the tendinous portion of the gastrocnemius as it becomes the Achilles tendon. FHL is the flexor hallucis longus, and Ag is the anterior muscle group.

The *tibialis posterior* arises from the upper two-thirds of the interosseous membrane and from the bones on each side of the membrane. It inclines medially to reach the medial malleolus and passes posteriorly to it in a "sling" (see Fig. 1–18). It sends two-thirds of its tendon to insert on the navicular with some of the fibers extending to the first cuneiform (Fig. 1–39).

The *flexor digitorum longus* arises from the posterior surface of the tibia distal to the soleus line and from the fascia of the posterior tibialis. Its tendon crosses the posterior tibialis tendon. It attaches to the distal phalanx of the four lateral toes (see Fig. 1–23).

The *flexor hallucis longus* originates from the fibula, the tibialis posterior fascia, and the interosseous membrane to insert into the terminal phalanx of the great toe (see Fig. 1–23) passing between the two sesamoid bones that are within the

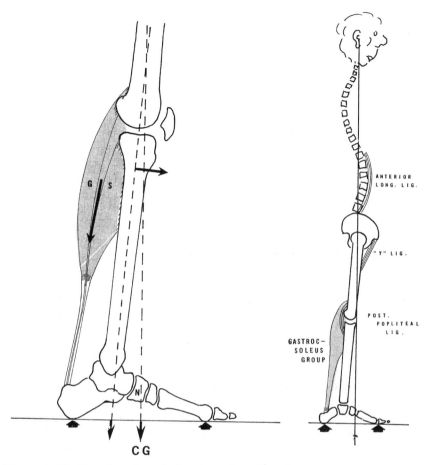

**Figure 1–37.** Muscular effort of relaxed two-legged standing position. In standing on both feet in a relaxed manner, the spine leans on the anterior longitudinal ligament, the hip on the iliofemoral (Y) ligament, and the knees extend to lean on the posterior popliteal ligaments. The gastrocnemius-soleus must maintain tonus to pull the leg back because the center of gravity falls some 3° ahead of the talus. Relaxed erect posture is principally ligamentous with only the gastrocnemius-soleus group active. (From Cailliet, R.: Low Back Pain Syndrome, ed. 3. F.A. Davis, 1968, with permission.)

tendons of the flexor hallucis brevis. It also sends fibrous slips to the tendons of the flexor digitorum longus as they pass to the second and third digits (Fig. 1–40).

## TERMINOLOGY

Ankle motion essentially consists of flexion and extension.[2] The definition of these terms regarding the foot and ankle, however, vary. The term *flexion*

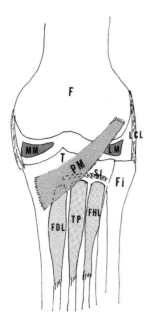

**Figure 1–38.** Plantaris muscle. The plantaris muscle (PM) originates from the lateral epicondyle of the femur (F) to attach upon the posterior superior aspect of the tibia (T). It runs laterally between the lateral collateral ligament (LCL) and the lateral meniscus (LM). The medial meniscus (MM) is noted, as is the head of the fibula (Fi). The three bipennate muscles—flexor digitorum longus (FDL), tibialis posterior (TP), and flexor hallucis longus (FHL)—originate below the site of attachment of the soleus muscle (SI).

usually implies that the angle between the two involved bones narrows, and *extension* indicates elongation or straightening, that is, increasing the angle. Some imply that the upward motion of the foot on the tibia should be extension because motion of the toes on the foot is also termed extension. The opposite therefore should be termed flexion.

Neurologically, upward movement of the foot is a part of the flexor synergy, as are hip and knee flexion. Currently, downward motion is termed *plantar flexion* and upward motion *dorsiflexion* as regards the foot-ankle complex.

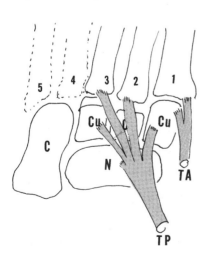

**Figure 1–39.** Tendinous attachment of the tibialis posterior tendon. The tibialis posterior (TP) tendon has two thirds of its attachment upon the navicular (N) with a slip to the first cuneiform (Cu), second and third metatarsal bones. Some fibers may connect to the cuboid (C). The tibial anterior tendon (TA) inserts upon the medial cuneiform and the base of the first metatarsal.

All the tendons passing behind the malleoli are considered plantar flexors. Medially, these are the tibialis posterior, flexor digitorum longus, and flexor hallucis longus. Laterally, these muscles are the peroneus longus and peroneus brevis, but these produce only approximately 5% of the total pull used to lift the heel off the ground. The major plantar flexor is the gastocnemius-soleus group.

Another term is that the motion of the foot-ankle complex occurs at the *joints of the ankle*.[3,4] The *ankle* is the junction between the tibia and the talus (within the mortise), that is, the *tibiotalar joint*. The *inferior* joint is the *subtalar joint*, about which occurs inversion-eversion and pronation-supination, which are subserved by the laterally and medially placed tendons.

## THE PLANTAR FASCIA

The plantar fascia is a continuation of the plantaris tendon. It originates from the medial tubercle of the calcaneus and proceeds anteriorly to split into five bands, with each attaching to a digit (Fig. 1–41). Each distal band splits at the metatarsophalangeal joint to attach to the inner and outer sides of the joint. Through this split pass the long and short flexor tendons (Fig. 1–42). There is frequently a short fibrous band that projects from the lateral aspect of the calcaneal tubercle and attaches to the base of the fifth metatarsal, forming part of the lateral "spring" ligament.

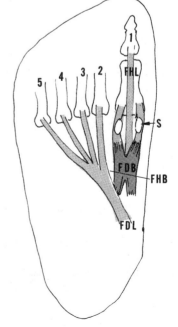

**Figure 1–40.** Tendinous attachment of the flexor hallucis longus and brevis. The flexor hallucis longus tendon (FHL) passes between the two sesamoid bones (S) present within the tendons of the flexor hallucis brevis (FHB) to attach to the base of the first (1) distal phalanx. The flexor digitorum longus (FDL) attaches into the bases of the second, third, fourth, and fifth digits.

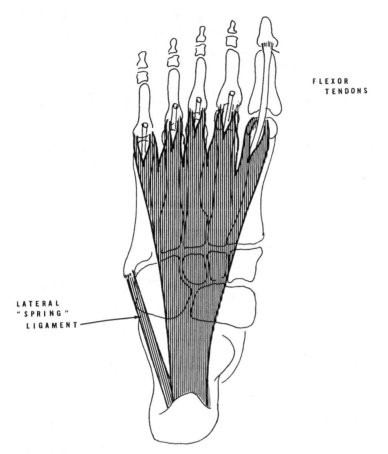

FLEXOR
TENDONS

LATERAL
"SPRING"
LIGAMENT

**Figure 1–41.** Plantar fascia. The plantar fascia originates from the calcaneal tuberosity. Passing anteriorly, it splits at each metatarsophalangeal joint to permit passage of the flexor tendons. A fibrous lateral band proceeds forward, attaching to the base of the fifth metatarsal, forming part of the lateral "spring" ligament.

## NERVE SUPPLY

The nerves to the muscles of the lower leg, ankle, and foot supply sensation and, hence, mediate pain, and supply motor function to the lower leg, foot, toes, and ankle. The major lower-extremity nerves are the branches of the sciatic nerve, which divides at the popliteal angle to form the tibial and common peroneal nerve (Fig. 1–43).

The *sciatic nerve* originates from undivided primary rami L4, L5, S1, S2, and S3.[4] It is a single trunk that divides into two components: the tibial and common peroneal nerves. These ultimately divide into branches that have various synonyms (Fig. 1–44).

The *tibial nerve*, which is essentially a continuation of the sciatic nerve, derives from all the undivided anterior primary rami of the sacral plexus. After it separates from the common peroneal nerve, it enters the lower leg between the origin of the two heads of the gastrocnemius muscle and then passes deep to the soleus muscle to enter the posterior compartment of the leg.

En route, the tibial nerve supplies both heads of the gastrocnemius muscle, the soleus, the plantaris, and the posterior tibialis muscle. It contributes to the formation of the sural nerve (see Fig. 1–46), which pierces the deep fascia of the middle third of the leg and then continues downward to form the *lateral calcaneal nerve*, which supplies the heel (Fig. 1–45).

The *posterior tibial nerve* is a continuation of the tibial nerve. It starts at the level of the fibrous arch of the soleus, courses downward on the tibia, and then terminates (under the flexor retinaculum, behind and inferior to the medial malleolus) into medial and lateral divisions of the plantar nerve (Fig. 1–46).

The *common peroneal nerve* is a comparatively short nerve containing segments of roots L4, L5, S1, and S2. It courses downward along the lateral border of the popliteal fossa to reach the head of the fibula posteriorly. It winds around the neck of the fibula, where it divides into the deep and superficial peroneal nerves.

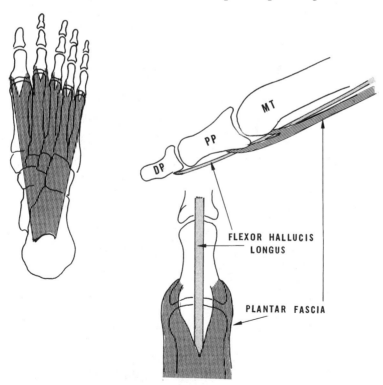

**Figure 1–42.** Anterior portion of the plantar fascia. The anterior splits in the plantar fascia (see Fig. 1–41) show the passage of the flexor tendons.

The *superficial peroneal nerve* descends down the leg in front of the fibula. Two-thirds down the lower leg it pierces the fascia and skin supplying the skin of the front, lateral side of the lower leg, and the dorsum of the foot.

The *deep peroneal nerve* begins just below the head of the fibula. After winding around the neck of the fibula, it descends the lower leg in front of the interosseous membrane. On reaching the ankle, it passes under the superior extensor retinaculum (see Fig. 1–34), where it divides into two branches, medial and lateral, to the skin surface of the lateral aspect of the great toe and second toe. Its motor function is to the extensor digitorum brevis, tibialis anterior, extensor hallucis longus, peroneus tertius, and first dorsal interosseous.

The *plantar nerves* are divisions of the posterior tibial nerve (see Fig. 1–46). The *medial plantar nerve* (Fig. 1–47) sends cutaneous sensory branches to the plantar surface of the medial three toes and the medial aspect of the fourth toe. Its motor branches supply the abductor hallucis, flexor hallucis brevis, flexor digitorum brevis, and the first two lumbricales (see Fig. 1–47).

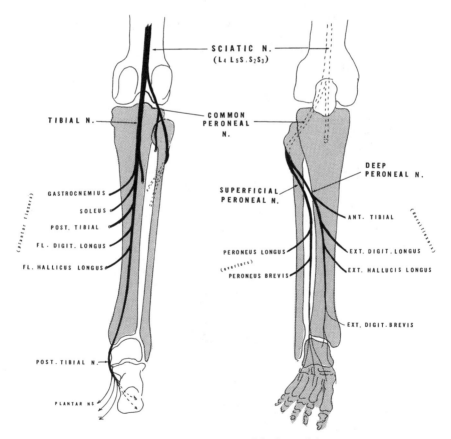

**Figure 1–43.** Innervation of the leg and foot.

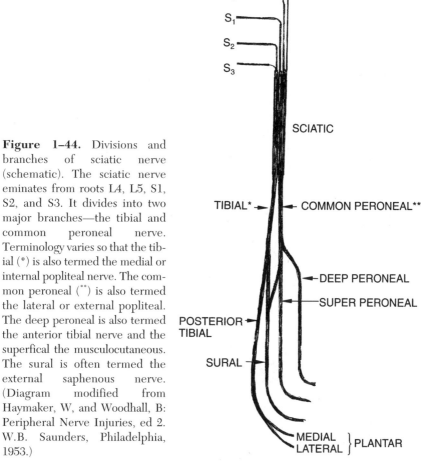

**Figure 1–44.** Divisions and branches of sciatic nerve (schematic). The sciatic nerve eminates from roots L4, L5, S1, S2, and S3. It divides into two major branches—the tibial and common peroneal nerve. Terminology varies so that the tibial (°) is also termed the medial or internal popliteal nerve. The common peroneal (°°) is also termed the lateral or external popliteal. The deep peroneal is also termed the anterior tibial nerve and the superfical the musculocutaneous. The sural is often termed the external saphenous nerve. (Diagram modified from Haymaker, W, and Woodhall, B: Peripheral Nerve Injuries, ed 2. W.B. Saunders, Philadelphia, 1953.)

The *lateral plantar nerve* passes across the plantar surface of the foot and, after dividing into deep and superficial branches, supplies the sensation of the plantar surface of the remaining toes on the lateral aspect of the foot. It supplies the motor innervation to the quadratus plantae, flexor digiti quinti brevis, abductor digiti quinti, and the remaining plantar interosseous and lumbrical muscles.

## BLOOD SUPPLY

The *popliteal artery* is a direct continuation of the femoral artery, which passes into the posterior popliteal quadrant and divides into the anterior and posterior tibial arteries going below the knee. The posterior tibial artery follows

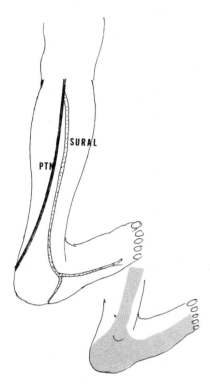

**Figure 1–45.** Sural nerve divisions and distribution.

the same course as the tibial nerve (Fig. 1–48) supplying the posterior muscles of the leg. On reaching the medial malleolus, it passes to the plantar surface of the foot, dividing into the medial and lateral plantar arteries. Below the bifurcation, the popliteal artery branches laterally, passing across the interosseous membrane, and then descends the lateral aspect of the leg supplying the lateral muscles. It ends as the *lateral calcaneal artery*.

Below the popliteal quadrant, the popliteal artery bifurcates, giving rise to the *anterior tibial artery*, which passes anteriorly between the tibia and fibula across the upper margin of the interosseous membrane, coursing down the anterior surface of the membrane where it supplies the muscles of the anterior compartment. On reaching the dorsum of the foot, it becomes the dorsalis pedis artery, whose terminal branches are the *dorsal metatarsal* and *dorsal digital* arteries. These communicate with the plantar distal branches of the plantar arteries (Fig. 1–49).

## LIGAMENTOUS STRUCTURE AND FUNCTION

Because ligaments are so important to the structure and function of the ankle and foot, a discussion of *ligaments* is warranted to understand function and impairment.

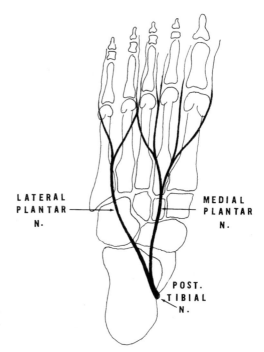

**Figure 1–46.** Division of the posterior tibial nerve into plantar nerves.

Dense connective tissue, which is the basis of tendons and ligaments, is a complex of cells, ground substance, and fibers. The fibers include collagen, elastin, and reticulum. The proportion of each of these fiber components is determined in the ultimate structure needed for a specific organ and function.

The basic building block of the collagen fiber is the *tropocollagen* molecule (Fig. 1–50). This molecule is a three-polypeptide chain attached together forming a collagen fiber. In the trihelix chain of amino acids, every third residue is glycine (Fig. 1–51). Each chain is of a uniform length and fits together with other chains in a precise configuration.

A *tendon* is a band of longitudinal collagen fibers attached to related articular areas at their periosteum to support an active and specific joint. Collagen fibers react to mechanical elongation in a specific manner. Their resulting length and tension form a *stress-strain curve*. Tendons are usually enclosed within a sheath having an intrinsic blood supply (Fig. 1–52).

*Stress* refers to the amount of tension (load) per unit cross-sectional area. *Strain* is the proportional elongation that occurs.

There are five distinct regions of collagen in the *stress-strain curve*[5]:

1. *Toe region*. There is very little increase in strain (length) from stress.
2. *Linear region*. Stiffness is basically consistent. As elongation increases, so does stress, and it is in this region that microfailure occurs early.

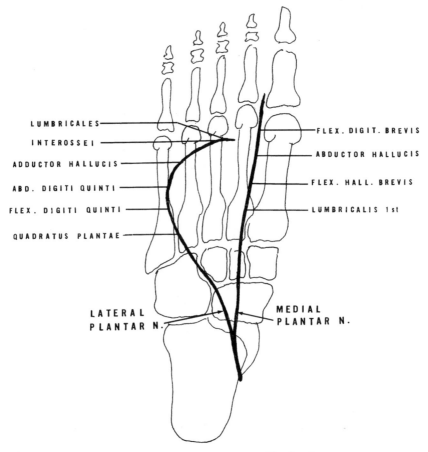

**Figure 1–47.** Muscles of the foot innervated by the plantar nerves.

3. *Progressive failure.* Although intact to the naked eye, a gradual failure occurs with progressive repeated strain.
4. *Major failure.* The tendon remains grossly intact, but there are points of shear and visible failure.
5. *Complete rupture region.* Gross tendon break.

## Creep

*Creep* is the slow elongation of a tendon in response to constant or repeated stress. Creep is transient if it is physiologic and under specific temperature variables.

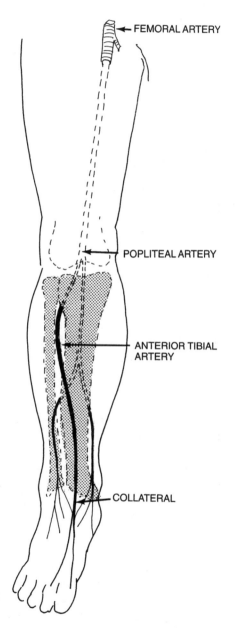

**Figure 1–48.** Arterial supply to the lower extremity.

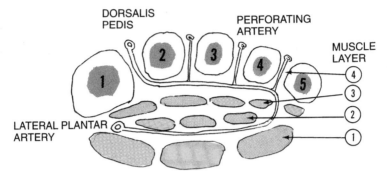

**Figure 1–49.** Distal blood supply of the foot. The lateral plantar artery passes medially between the first (1) and second layers (2) of the muscles of the sole of the foot to then move laterally under the metatarsal and the fourth layer of intrinsic muscles (not shown in figure). The arterial supply ends at the dorsalis pedis artery with intermediate perforating arteries.

## Recovery

*Recovery* is the return of a tendon to its original length following removal of the stress prior to rupture. If stress is removed before partial failure, the tendon will return to its original length after a period of rest during which there is no load. This is termed *recovery*. This recovery is dependent on the previous stress and the time of recovery. Previous gentle stretching changes the curve by a significant degree.[6]

Recovery does not imply that there has been no residual permanent damage, nor that there has not been permanent elongation. Recovery of one function does not imply recovery of all other functions, because microfailure may persist.

Stress is a physical stimulus that plays a significant role in the formation and maintenance of collagen. A gradual increase in stress increases the production and organization of collagen. A decrease in stress causes a decrease in collagen production and organization.

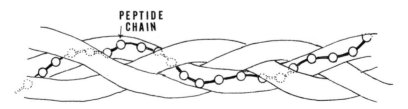

**Figure 1–50.** Type I collagen molecule.

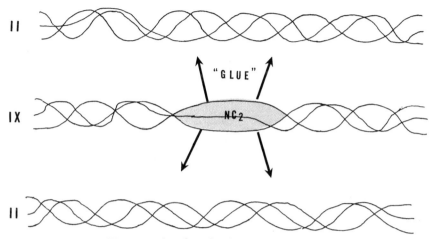

**Figure 1–51.** The role of type IX in cartilage.

Injury to collagen structures results in scar formation. After injury there is cell migration from the wound edges into the space formed. Initially macrophages are followed by fibroblasts. These form around blood vessels with original capillaries becoming blood vessels. Leukocytes also invade, and in 48 to 72 hours, collagen fibers emerge. Either acute trauma or repetitive chronic irritants always initiate an inflammatory reaction with ultimate fibroplasia. How microphages stimulate fibroplasia remains unclear.

In nontraumatized tissue, significant changes in the compliance, strength, and elongation of dense connective tissues (DCT) occur:

1. Immobilization causes a significant loss of strength. A loss of 80% in DCT strength in muscle has been found after 4 weeks, 50% in collateral ligaments, and 39% in cruciate ligaments of the knee after 8 weeks.[7]
2. Immobilization causes a loss of length and flexibility more slowly than loss of strength.

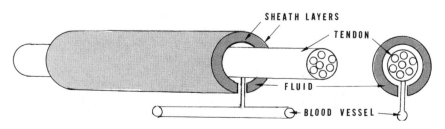

**Figure 1–52.** Tendon sheath and blood supply.

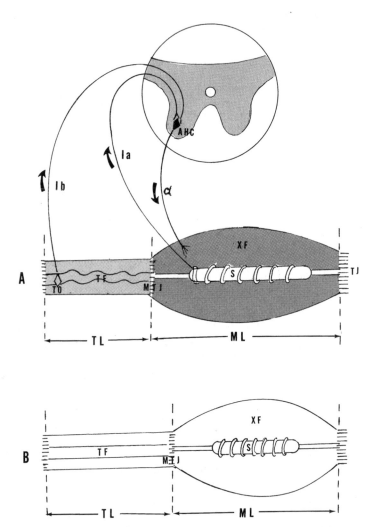

**Figure 1–53.** Musculotendinous mechanism. (A) The spindle system (S) measures the length of the muscle (ML), and the tendon organs (Golgi) (TO) monitor the tension. Stretching the spindle system activates the Ia fiber, whereas stretching the tendon organ activates the Ib fibers. These influence the anterior horn cells (AHC), which send motor fiber activity via the alpha fibers to the extrafusal fibers (XF). With the muscle at resting level (A), the tendon fibers (TF) are slightly coiled. When the extrafusal fibers contract (B), the muscle (ML) shortens, and the tendon elongates (TL) to the degree that the tendon fibers can elongate. The tendon fibrils (TF) composed of collagen fibers uncoil. Excessive muscle contraction can tear the muscle-tendon juncture (MTJ).

3. Trauma prior to immobilization accelerates shortening of DCT during immobilization because of scar formation.

4. Overuse of injuries may be prevented or minimized by periods of rest between stress.

5. Contracture may be prevented or minimized by placing DCT structures in a lengthened position during immobilization.

6. Isometric muscular contractions initiate prophylactic stress to tendons.

## SENSORY MECHANISMS OF TENDONS AND LIGAMENTS

Orthopedic literature has been largely devoted to bony, ligamentous, and vascular anatomy with little attention paid to articular neuronal structures. Neuronal structures have been considered as mostly subserving pain mechanisms and providing "ligamentomuscular protective reflexes." These latter reflexes were considered to constitute a fast feedback system preventing abnormal joint movements. Several authors have recently realized that no reflex is fast enough to reflexly protect the joint unless the threatened trauma is quite slow.[8] Joint receptors must therefore subserve other functions.

Numerous sensory nerve endings within tendons and ligaments have afferent fibers to the gamma muscle spindles that allegedly stabilize joints and prevent traumatic excesses to their soft tissues.[9] The proprioceptive function of many joints has been studied: finger,[10–12] elbow,[13] knee,[14,15] and hip.[16] However, few studies of the foot and ankle[17,18] have been performed.

A number of peripheral sensory receptors have been proposed as being able to signal limb position and movement, including joint capsular, muscle spindle, and cutaneous receptors.[19] Proprioceptive reception is dependent on the age of the subject,[11] the amplitude and velocity of the motion,[10] and whatever receptors are responsible (Fig. 1–53).[17]

## REFERENCES

1. Basmajian, JV: Grant's Method of Anatomy, ed 4. Williams & Wilkins, Baltimore, 1971, pp 404–416.
2. American Academy of Orthopaedic Surgeons: Joint Motion—Method of Measuring and Recording. American Academy of Orthopaedic Surgeons, Rosemont, IL, 1965.
3. Inman, VT: The Joints of the Ankle. Williams & Wilkins, Baltimore, 1976, pp 26–29.
4. Haymaker, W, and Woodhall, B: Peripheral Nerve Injuries: Principles of Diagnosis, ed 2. WB Saunders, Philadelphia, 1953, pp 286–293.
5. Tillman, LJ, and Cummings, GS: Biological Mechanisms of Connective Tissue Mutability. In Currier, DP, and Nelson, RM (eds): Dynamics of Human Biological Tissues. FA Davis, Philadelphia, 1992, Chap 1, pp 1–44.
6. Rigby, BJ, Hirai, N, and Spikes, JD: The mechanical behavior of rat tail tendon. J Gen Physiol 43:265–283, 1959.

7. Cummings, GS, and Tillman, LJ: Remodeling of dense connective tissue in normal adult tissues. In Currier, DP, and Nelson, RM (eds): Dynamics of Human Biological Tissues. FA Davis, Philadelphia, 1992, Chap 2, pp 45–73.

8. Wright, V, and Radin, EL (eds): Mechanics of Human Joints: Physiology, Pathophysiology and Treatment. Marcel Dekker, New York, 1993.

9. Johansson, H, Lorentzon, R, Sjolander, P, and Sojka, P: The anterior cruciate ligament: A sensor action on the gamma-muscle-spindle systems of muscles around the knee joint. Neuro-Orthop 9:1–23, 1990.

10. Clark, FJ, Grigg, P, and Chapin, JW: The contribution of articular receptors to proprioception with fingers in human. J Neurophysiol 61:186–193, 1989.

11. Ferrell, WR, Crighton, A, and Sturrock, RD: Age-dependent changes in position sense in human proximal interphalangeal joints. Neuro Report 3:259–261, 1992.

12. Ferrel, WR, Crighton, A, and Sturrock, RD: Position sense at the proximal interphalangeal joint is distorted in patients with rheumatoid arthritis of finger joints. Exp Physiol 77:675–680, 1992.

13. Goodwin, GM, McCloskey, DI, and Matthews, PBC: The contribution of muscle afferents to kinaesthesia shown by vibrating induced illusions of movement and by the effects of paralyzing joint afferents. Brain 95:705–748, 1972.

14. Barrack, RL, Skinner, HB, Cook, SD, and Haddad, RJ: Effect of articular disease and total knee arthroplasty on knee joint-position sense. J Neurophysiol 50:684–687, 1983.

15. Horch, KW, Clark, FJ, and Burgess, PR: Awareness of knee joint angle under static conditions. J Neurophysiol 38:1436–1447, 1975.

16. Grigg, P, Finerman, GA, and Riley, LH: Joint position sense after total hip replacement. J Bone Joint Surg 55-A:1016–1025, 1973.

17. Freeman, MR, and Wyke, B: The innervation of the ankle joint: An anatomical and histological study in the cat. J Anat 68:321–333, 1967.

18. Freeman, MAR, and Wyke, B: Articular reflexes in the ankle joint: An electromyographic study of normal and abnormal influences of ankle-joint mechanoreceptors upon reflex activity in the leg muscles. Br J Surg 54:990–1001, 1967.

19. Hall, MG, Ferrell, WR, Baxendale, RH, and Hamblen, DL: Knee joint proprioception: Threshold detection levels in healthy young subjects. Neuro-Orthop 15:81–90, 1994.

# CHAPTER 2

# The Walking Foot: Gait

To understand the role of the foot and ankle, all of the components of gait must be analyzed.[1] Walking is the human being's means of moving from one site to another. It demands free and full range of motion of all involved joints, adequate coordinated neuromuscular activity, and energy conservation. Observations on the mechanics of walking were recorded as far back as Aristotle and Leonardo da Vinci, but recently, walking has been studied scientifically in a three-dimensional manner by the combined use of cameras, mirrors, and electromyography.[2] More recently, pressure transducer mats have been informative.

There are many terms that have evolved in the study of the mechanics of locomotion,[2] many of which merit definition:

1. *Kinematics*. Outcome measurements including displacement, velocity, and acceleration.
2. *Kinetics*. Outcome measurements including the forces and movements that produce the motion.
3. *Ground reaction forces*. The reaction force on all body segments imposed by the ground during the stance phase. This mass-acceleration consists of three vectors: one vertical and two shear. The vertical force can equal 1.5 to 2.0 times the body weight.
4. *Center of pressure*. This is the center of force in the vertical vector acting on the foot during stance. It is *not* the center of gravity.
5. *Joint moment*. This is the torque (moment) of forces, active and passive, on joints during rotation about its axis.
6. *Joint reaction force*. The force of reaction between the two segments of a moving joint.
7. *Mechanical stress*. Measurement of force per unit area.

8. *Moment of inertia.* The resistance to rotation as related to the axis about which there is rotation. Where considered pertinent, any of these terms will be further discussed.

Human locomotion has been compared to a wheel rolling over the ground with two spokes being the legs. The spoke that touches the ground constitutes the *stance* and the spoke that moves, the *swing* phase

Gait begins with movement from the initial stance when both feet are on the floor, but not as a double-limb support because there need not necessarily be equal weight bearing on both legs (Fig. 2–1). Single-limb support is more appropriate since the weight (center of gravity) shifts laterally until there is one-leg stance (support). The percentage of the gait related to stance, double and single leg, has been mathematically computed (Fig. 2–2).

Walking is initiated by inclining the body forward, placing it ahead of its center of gravity. The body also simultaneously shifts its weight laterally, placing more weight on the stance foot. As the center of gravity changes, one leg must be brought forward ahead of the other and of the shifted center of gravity to prevent falling forward.

Gait is divided into two phases: *stance* and *swing*, with stance being 60% and swing 40%.[3,4] The leg that moves forward to regain balance is termed the *swing limb*. The leg that maintains balance is the *stance leg*. The stance phase begins when the swing-leg heel strikes the floor ahead of the body (Fig. 2–3). The precise duration of these gait cycles varies with the walking velocity, so that total stance and swing times shorten as the gait velocity increases.

## GAIT DETERMINANTS

If an individual were to walk with knees stiff and pelvis moving in a straight line, his or her center of gravity would describe a high, undulating pathway (Fig. 2–4) with a high expenditure of energy. Its highest point would occur when the

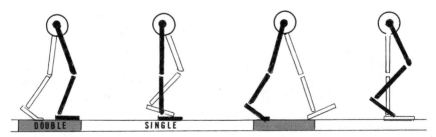

**Figure 2–1.** Division of floor contact during gait. Initially a person stands on both legs (double), but as one leg swings, there is a single-leg balance in the stance phase. There are three intervals of the single to the double phase.

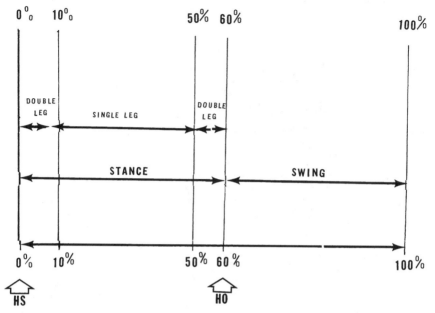

**Figure 2–2.** Percentage of gait divided into stance and swing.

stiff weight-bearing leg was vertical (midstance) and its lowest when one limb was fully flexed and the other extended at the hip yet both weight bearing (see third figure of double stance in Fig. 2–1) (Fig. 2–5).

Besides being energy-demanding, this gait would be jerky by alternately elevating and depressing the body weight at each step. Human beings do not normally walk in this manner but use various movements of the hip, knees, ankles, and pelvis to maintain the center of gravity (Fig. 2–6) on a horizontal plane. These movements, which are termed *determinants of gait*,[5,6] increase efficiency, decrease the expenditure of energy, and make gait more graceful.

During a complete cycle of gait, the center of gravity is displaced twice in its vertical axis. The high peak is during the middle of stance phase, when the weight-bearing leg is extended and vertical, and the low peak is at heel strike, when the hind leg is at toe-off and both legs are weight-bearing. The undulating center of gravity may transcribe a cycle with a vertical displacement of 2 inches.

The determinants of gait that decrease this degree of displacement are discussed in the following sections.

## Pelvic Rotation

During walking, the pelvis rotates about an axis located at the lumbosacral spine. Viewed from above (Fig. 2–7), one side of the pelvis comes forward with

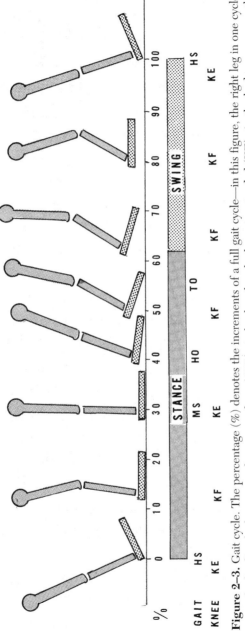

**Figure 2–3.** Gait cycle. The percentage (%) denotes the increments of a full gait cycle—in this figure, the right leg in one cycle. HS is the heel strike beginning the stance phase (62%). At heel strike, the knee is extended (KE). As the body passes over the weight-bearing leg, the knee flexes slightly (KF) to absorb the shock. At midstance (MS 30%), the knee again is fully extended (KE). At heel off (HO 40%), the knee begins to flex slightly (KF 50%) and remains flexed through toe off (TO 62%) when the swing phase begins. The knee remains flexed throughout the swing phase until just before heel strike recurs, when the knee re-extends (KE 100%). (From Cailliet, R: Knee Pain and Disability, ed 2. FA Davis, Philadelphia, 1983, Fig. 113, p 154, with permission.)

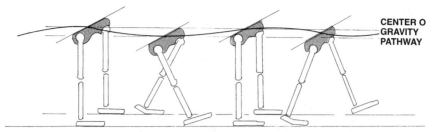

**Figure 2–4.** Undulating course of pelvic center in gait without determinants. This figure shows the marked vertical undulations of the center of gravity that occur when gait is performed with stiff knees and no lateral or vertical movement of the pelvis.

the limb that is swinging forward. As the pelvis rotates, the angle between the pelvis and the thigh lessens, as does the angle between the leg and the floor (Fig. 2–8). The pelvis rotates approximately 4° on each side for a total rotation of 8°. From this rotation, the vertical undulation of the center of gravity decreases three-eighths of an inch.

## Pelvic Tilt

Pelvic tilting is another determinant of gait that decreases the degree of undulation (Fig. 2–9). During gait, the pelvis drops on the side where the leg

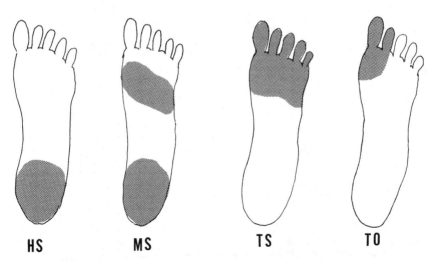

HS        MS        TS        TO

**Figure 2–5.** Foot support during stance phase. As shown by F-scan sensor mappings, the pressure areas of the foot during heel strike (HS), midstance (MS), and terminal stance (TS) before toe off (TO) are shown.

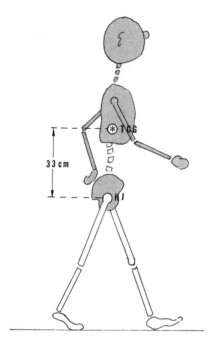

**Figure 2–6.** The thoracic center of gravity. The thoracic center of gravity (TCG) is anterior to the 10th thoracic vertebra and approximately 33 cm above the hip joint (HJ).

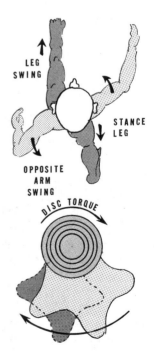

**Figure 2–7.** Pelvic and lumbar vertebral rotation during gait. During gait, the pelvis rotates as part of the determinants. In addition to disk torque, the swing phase of the lower extremity alternates with contralateral arm swings. (From Cailliet, R: Low Back Pain Syndrome, ed 5, 1994, FA Davis, Philadelphia, Fig. 10-22, p 281, with permission.)

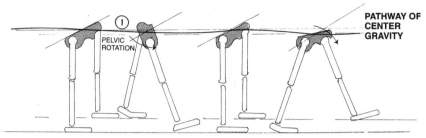

**Figure 2–8.** Pelvic rotation: A determinant of gait. The pelvis rotates forward with the "swinging" leg, thus decreasing the angle formed by the leg with the floor and at the hip joint. This rotation decreases the vertical undulations of the center of gravity of the pelvis.

swings. During this phase, the stance leg is slightly adducted into a Trendelenberg position and the swing leg slightly abducted. The swing leg flexes at the hip and knee to clear the floor. The adducted position of the stance leg decreases the vertical undulation an additional one-eighth of an inch.

## Pelvic Shift

As one walks, the pelvis moves laterally to maintain balance as one leg is lifted from the ground to swing. This rhythmic, lateral sway maintains balance but also smooths the pelvic movement during gait.

The combination of pelvic rotation, pelvic tilting, and pelvic shift significantly decreases the degree of undulation (Fig. 2–10).

## Knee Flexion during Stance

During the stance phase, the knee that has been extended at heel strike flexes. It flexes approximately 15° as the body moves over its center of gravity, then gradually re-extends at the end of stance phase (Fig. 2–11).

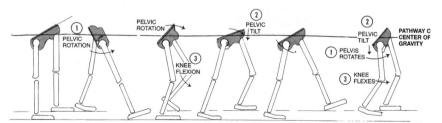

**Figure 2–9.** Pelvic tilt: Second determinant of gait. Pelvic rotation has been discussed (1). As the left leg swings through, the pelvis on the left drops (2) and the left hip and knee flex. The last figure on the right shows the right leg swinging through with the right side of the pelvis dipping and the right hip and knee flexing.

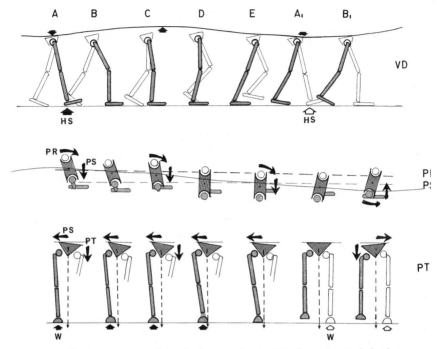

**Figure 2–10.** Composition of determinants of gait. VD shows vertical displacement from the side view. PR is pelvic rotation as the leg swings through. PT indicates pelvic tilt. The bottom figure illustrates gait from the front and shows lateral shift of the pelvis combined with tilt and rotation. The weight-bearing leg (W) goes into a Trendelenburg position, that is, adducting as the pelvis shifts over it. The swinging leg is slightly abducted. PS indicates pelvic shift and the arrows the direction of the shift.

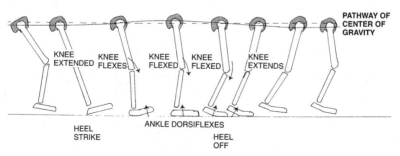

**Figure 2–11.** Knee flexion during stance phase of gait: Third determinant. The knee is fully extended at heel strike. As the body moves over the center of gravity, the knee flexes to decrease the vertical amplitude of the pathway of the center of gravity. This slight flexion also cushions the impact on the body. The knee re-extends at the end of the stance phase: the "heel off."

## Knee-Ankle Relationship During Gait

As the knee flexes and re-extends, a foot-ankle-knee relationship occurs which influences the degree of pelvic undulation. At heel strike, the foot-ankle is dorsiflexed to 90°. There is gradual plantar flexion as the foot becomes flat on the ground during midstance when the body is directly above the foot.

As the ankle joint passes over the weight-bearing heel (Fig. 2–12), two small arcs of motion occur. These are "smoothed" out by the slight knee flexion (Fig. 2–13). The anterior tibialis decelerates the foot from active contraction at heel strike to flat foot during the stance phase. The quadriceps, contracted at heel strike with the knee fully extended, decelerates the knee flexion at midstance (Fig. 2–14).

During each gait cycle, the ankle travels through four arcs of motion.[7-9] The ankle alternately dorsiflexes and plantar flexes, with the first three arcs occurring during the stance phase and the fourth during swing phase. Each averages 30° (between 20 and 40°).

All of the determinants of gait allegedly decrease the degree of vertical undulation, thus decreasing the energy expenditure and also smoothing the gait. The speed of locomotion is dependent on the length of the stride and the increase in cadence. The determinants of gait improve the forward velocity without increasing cadence, thus improving the energy requirement.

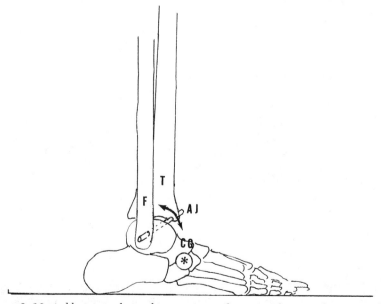

**Figure 2–12.** Ankle joint relationship to center of gravity. The axis of rotation of the ankle joint (AJ) is posterior to the center of gravity (CG) of the foot. The heel lever arm is shorter than the forefoot lever arm; hence, there is rotation at the hind forefoot (°).

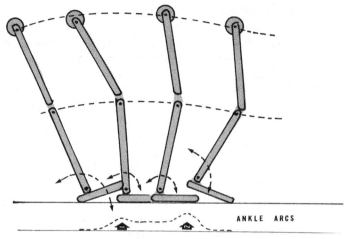

**Figure 2–13.** Foot-ankle relationship in gait: Fourth determinant. At heel strike the ankle is dorsiflexed 90° (and supinated). The level of the ankle rises slightly as the foot goes forward into the "flatfoot stance." This is followed by the ankle again dorsiflexing as the leg passes over the foot. At push-off the heel rises, giving a second small upward undulation. These small undulations at the ankle are "smoothed out" by simultaneous knee flexions.

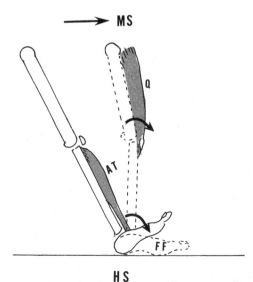

**Figure 2–14.** Anterior tibialis and quadriceps deceleration. At heel strike (HS), the anterior tibialis (AT) is contracted to dorsiflex the foot. The quadriceps (Q) is also contracted to keep the knee extended. As the body comes (straight arrow) to midstance (MS), the anterior tibialis decelerates the foot plantar flexion until it becomes flat to the ground (FF). The knee flexes slightly as the quadriceps decelerates the knee flexion (curved arrow).

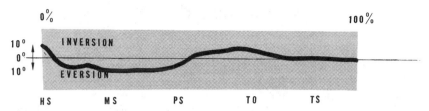

**Figure 2–15.** Subtalar joint motion during walking. In evaluating inversion and eversion of the foot in the percentage of gait cycle (100%), it is estimated as 10° of either at heel strike (HS), midstance (MS), preswing (PS) and toe-off (TO), ending at terminal stance (TS).

## ROTATIONAL DETERMINANTS OF GAIT

The above determinants have been discussed in the sagittal plane of the lower extremities other than pelvic "rotation," but there are also lower-extremity rotational aspects of gait occurring in the thigh, lower leg, ankle, and foot.

As the limb begins its swing phase, the femur gradually rotates internally with the tibia also simultaneously rotating inwardly on the femur. This rotation continues past the heel strike into the stance phase and ends when the foot is fully flat on the ground surface at midstance. At this point in the gait, the opposite leg begins its swing phase and its internal rotation.

On reaching the flat-foot stance at midstance phase, the pelvis begins derotation of the weight-bearing limb. The hip and lower leg gradually rotate externally. Because the foot is weight-bearing and thus "fixed" on the ground, rotation of the foot must occur at the subtalar joint (Fig. 2–15) because no rotation of the talus is possible within the ankle mortise.

In gait, the weight-bearing foot finds a normal "toe-out" of approximately 6 to 7° from the sagittal direction (Fig. 2–16). As a person ages, this toe-out increases to improve balance. In faster walking, stability is less a concern and the toe-out decreases to the point of being totally eliminated.

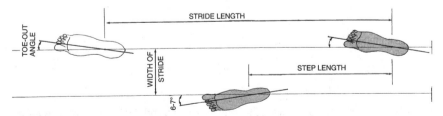

**Figure 2–16.** Outward angulation of the feet during walking. A toe-out angle of 6 to 7° is usual but increases with aging and decreases to 0° with an increase in pace. The length of stride is measured from an initial stance of the foot to the next stance of the same foot.

## SHOCK ABSORPTION

As the body weight transfers from swing phase, there is an abrupt impact at the heel strike: approximately 60% of the body weight within 0.02 seconds. The immediate reaction is plantar flexion, which is terminated by the deceleration action of the pretibial muscles.

The impact is also diminished by slight knee flexion, which is terminated by the deceleration effect of the quadriceps muscle group. The previously mentioned action of the anterior tibialis group actuates forward motion of the tibia, which initiates knee flexion.

## MUSCULAR ACTION OF GAIT

The trunk, hip, leg, foot, and ankle muscles activate all elements of gait for motion, stabilization, and deceleration. These muscles act across two or more joints as the extremity moves from a fixed point of stance to forward locomotion.

Walking actually begins with relaxation of the gastrocnemius-soleus muscle group, allowing forward inclination of the body ahead of the center of gravity (Fig. 2–17). With the anterior shift of body weight, the supporting foot becomes the *propulsive* foot, with its weight bearing shifting from the heel

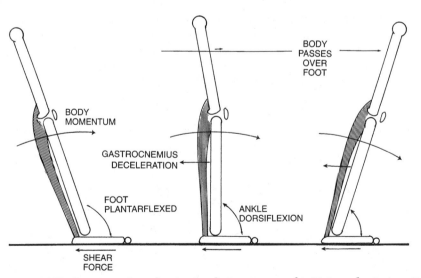

**Figure 2–17.** Gastrocnemius-soleus action during stance and initiation of gait. As gait begins the stance phase, the body momentum is forward and the foot plantar flexes. The gastrocnemius becomes engaged in decelerating the forward momentum. At midstance the gastrocnemius also assists in flexing the knee. As the body passes over the center before heel-off, there is further deceleration from the gastrocnemius muscle.

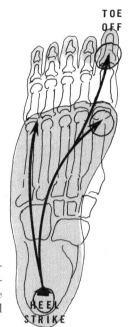

**Figure 2–18.** Path of weight bearing of the foot during walking. Weight bearing begins at the heel (*heel strike*) and proceeds along the lateral border of the foot toward the metatarsal heads with the major propulsive thrust by the distal phalanx of the big toe (*heel-off*).

along the lateral side of the foot, across the metatarsal heads toward the pad of the big toe (Fig. 2–18). The big toe then plantar-flexes against the ground, stabilizing the foot and assisting in ultimate push-off.

Major muscular activity begins during the last 10° of the swing phase and ends after the first 10° of the stance phase (Fig. 2–19). The muscular activity at the end of the swing phase is that of deceleration rather than forward propulsion (Fig. 2–20).

## THE FOOT-ANKLE COMPLEX IN GAIT

There are three major joint complexes in the foot that are involved in walking: the subtalar, the midtarsal, and the metatarsophalangeal (Fig. 2–21).

The subtalar joint (talocalcaneal) (see Fig. 1–8) is the joint between the calcaneus and the talus, which bears the weight of the body at the tibiotalar joint. It has a single, obliquely oriented axis, which allows the foot to tilt medially (inversion) and laterally (eversion), in both stance and swing phases of gait. Subtalar action is definitely related to rotation of the leg (Fig. 2–22).

The midtarsal joint (transverse tarsal joint) (see Fig. 1–13) is the junction between the hindfoot and the forefoot: the talonavicular and the calcaneocuboid joints. It forms a reasonably stable arch, which can flatten with liga-

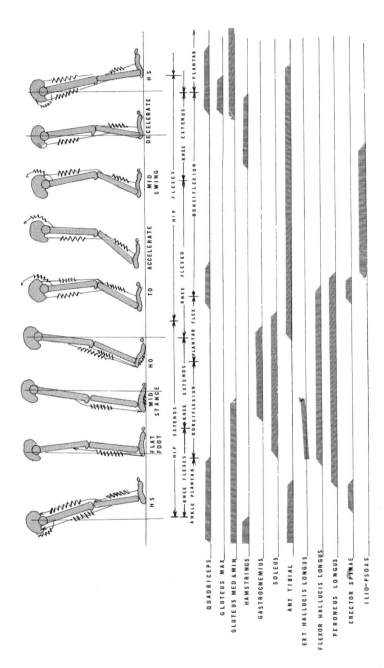

**Figure 2–19.** Muscular activities of normal walking. The various muscular groups related to the hip, knee, ankle, and foot motions throughout the various aspects of the gait cycle are depicted.

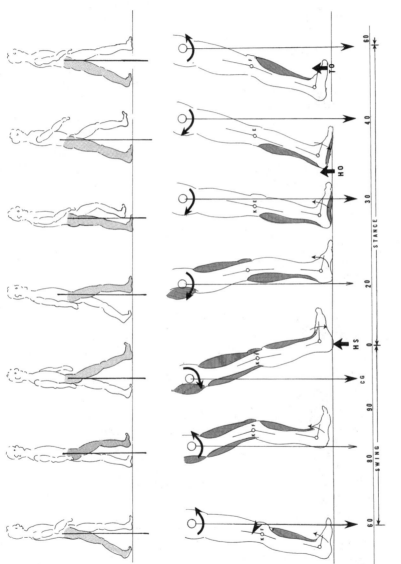

**Figure 2–20.** Muscular activities of the lower extremity during normal gait. The various muscular groups related to the hip, knee, ankle, and foot motions through a complete stride cycle in normal gait as viewed in the right leg are depicted.

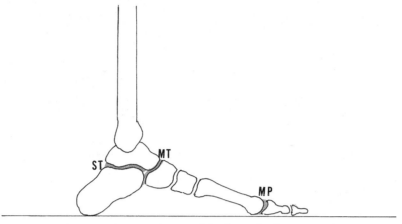

**Figure 2–21.** The major functional joints of the foot. The three major functional joints of the foot are as follows: ST = the subtalar; MT = the midtarsal; MP = the metatarsophalangeal.

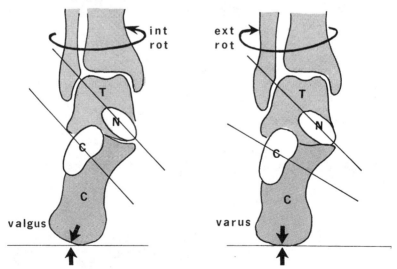

**Figure 2–22.** Supination of the foot during external rotation of the leg. With the foot weight bearing during the stance phase, external rotation of the leg causes the foot to rotate at the subtalar joint and supinate the foot. The leg begins to externally rotate during walking when the foot is fully flat against the ground. The supinated position places the calcaneus into more varus and thus places the Achilles tendon in a more direct alignment with the leg.

mentous laxity but flatten more in the longitudinal arch during dorsiflexion and plantar flexion. Its degree of mobility has not been measured.

The metatarsophalangeal (see Fig. 1–21) joints are the articulations between the five metatarsal heads and the proximal phalanges. At ankle dorsiflexion, these joints may also be at dorsiflexion, becoming neutral at midstance and dorsiflexed as much as 25° at toe-off. As the foot "pushes off," they remain in contact with the ground and act as plantar flexors.

## MUSCULAR CONTROL

Muscular control of the foot progresses from the hindfoot to the forefoot, and then to the toes (Fig. 2–23). There are 10 muscles involved. The subtalar joint is prominent, and thus the muscles involved are prominent and considered in groups.

---

Inverters
    Tibialis posterior
    Tibialis anterior
    Flexor digitorum longus
    Flexor hallucis longus
    Soleus
Everters
    Peroneus longus
    Peroneus brevis
    Extensor digitorum longus
    Extensor hallucis longus

---

The *inverters* cross the subtalar joint in a medial direction with all but the tibialis anterior lying posterior to the ankle The *everters* lie on the lateral side of the subtalar joint axis.

The foot also passively undergoes motion during other aspects of walking, such as stair climbing and descending (Figs. 2–24 and 2–25), that need examination during complete evaluation of the foot and ankle.

## FLOOR CONTACT

Contact with the ground has already been discussed, but as it is a valid concern in foot pain from abnormal gait from whatever cause, further consideration is paramount. This has encouraged surface forces studies.[10-15]

Heel pressure studies show two patterns (1) initial loading at the posterior lateral aspect of the foot, which occurs at the initial heel strike: 70% to 100% body weight, which occurs within 0.05 seconds[15,16]; and (2) at the big toe on push-off: usually 10%.

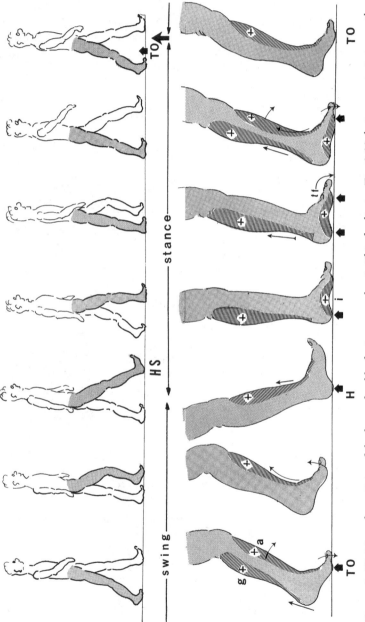

**Figure 2–23.** Muscular activity of the leg and ankle during normal gait. This duplicates Fig. 2-20, but concentrates upon the leg, ankle, and foot during gait from toe-off through a full stride.

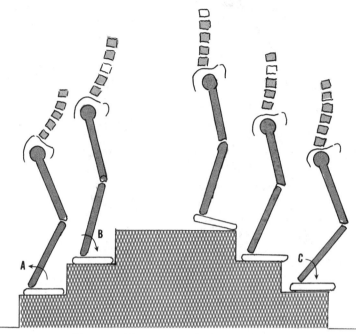

**Figure 2–24.** Foot-ankle action during stair climbing and descending. As a person climbs stairs, the knee flexes about 50% and the body leans forward. The foot-ankle initially dorsiflexes passively (A) and gradually plantar-flexes (B) as the knee extends. In descent, the gastrocnemius-soleus decelerates the foot as it dorsiflexes passively (C). (From Cailliet, R.: Knee Pain and Disability, ed 2. FA Davis, Philadelphia, 1983, Fig. 73, p 93, with permission.)

As the body moves ahead to midstance, the weight bearing of the heel reduces one-third,[16] and weight bearing increases more distally toward the metatarsal heads.

Metatarsal head pressures differ in each toe, with the highest pressures registered under the second and third metatarsals[12,14,17] (see Fig. 2–5), but this varies with individuals and in varying gaits.

Of the toes, the hallux sustains the greatest pressure, with the fifth the least.[16]

## ABNORMAL ANKLE-FOOT DEVIATIONS IN PATHOLOGIC GAITS

There are numerous abnormal gaits that develop with central and peripheral nervous diseases as well as with various orthopedic deformities. Each is discussed in subsequent sections as these pathologic conditions are discussed.

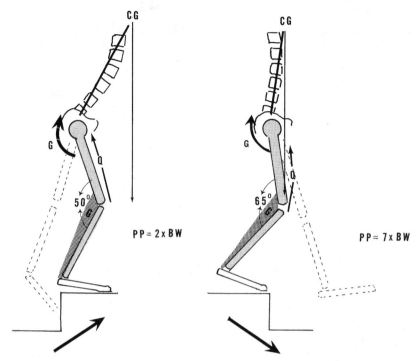

**Figure 2–25.** Stair climbing and descent. Besides the patellar pressure invoked in this activity, the knee to foot-ankle relationship is also involved. The figure to the left indicates a 50° knee flexion which changes the gastrocnemius muscle length while it is elongating to allow ankle dorsiflexion. The right figure indicates that at descent, the knee flexes 65°, which further lengthens the gastrocnemius muscle as it further decelerates ankle dorsiflexion. With a constant change in the relationship to the center of gravity (CG), the body weight alters vertical forces. (From Cailliet, R.: Knee Pain and Disability, ed 2. FA Davis, Philadelphia, 1983, Fig. 74 p 94, with permission.)

There are generally used terms that merit general discussion. *Equinus* is excessive plantar flexion with inadequate ankle dorsiflexion. *Drop foot* is excessive plantar flexion from inadequate active ankle dorsiflexion, usually caused by a flaccid neuromuscular condition. *Calcaneus* is excessive weight-bearing impact on the heel from excessive and uncontrolled ankle dorsiflexion.[1]

Faulty knee and hip function inevitably causes abnormal foot and ankle function during pathologic gait, which must be recognized as contributing to the foot-ankle impairment and the resultant disability.

A wide variety of foot and ankle disorders can be diagnosed with a new device that performs and records pressure mapping during gait. The device is a thin, flexible sensor that was originally developed for analyzing dental maloc-

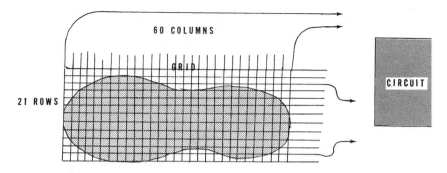

**Figure 2–26.** Pressure mapping system for gait analysis. The system consists of grids with silver-based rows and columns that are pressure sensitive. These record the pressure, timing, and differentiation as to heel, midfoot, and forefoot. The circuit generates a computer printout.

clusion. It contains nearly 1000 sensing locations over its surface. It can be trimmed to fit almost any shoe and yet permit full functionality.

By means of a computer, it records the tactile information. It is designed for installation in any IBM-compatible personal computer (PC) with VGA-level graphics support and a 40-megabyte hard drive.

Originally, gait studies were performed by testing with rigid triaxial force plates attached to video cameras mounted under glass windows to observe the human foot during gait. The sensor consists of a gridwork of rows and columns formed by silver-based, conductive ink deposition (Fig. 2–26), which is pressure sensitive. These sensations are transmitted via a coaxial cable to the rest of the electronics that display, store, and print the data collected.

The gait analysis system displays the foot in three sections—heel, midfoot, and forefoot. The pressure variants are displayed in color and are graded according to toe pressure distribution and time of the gait.°

## REFERENCES

1. Perry, J: Gait Analysis: Normal and Pathological Function. McGraw-Hill, New York, 1992.
2. Pathokinesiology Department, Physical Therapy Department: Observational Gait Analysis Handbook. Professional Staff Association of Rancho Los Amigos Medical Center, Downey, California, 1989.
3. Mann, R: Biomechanics. In Jahss, MH (ed): Disorders of the Foot, vol 1. WB Saunders, Philadelphia, 1982, pp 37–67.
4. Murray, MP, Drought, AB, and Kory, RC: Walking patterns of normal men. J Bone Joint Surg 46A(2):335–360, 1964.

---

°This equipment is currently manufactured by Tekscan, Inc., 451 D Street, 4th Floor, Boston, Massachusetts 02210.

5. Saunder, JB de CM, Inman, VT, and Eberhart, HD: The major determinants in normal and pathological gait. J Bone Joint Surg 35A:543, 1953.
6. Morton, DJ: Human Locomotion and Body Form: A Study of Gravity and Man. Williams & Wilkins, Baltimore, 1952.
7. Eberhart, HD, Inman, VT, and Bressler, B: The principle elements in human locomotion. In Klopsteg, PE, and Wilson, PD (eds): Human Limbs and Their Substitutes. Hafner, New York, 1968, pp 437–471.
8. Locke, M, Perry, J, Campbell, J, and Thomas, L: Ankle and subtalar motion during gait in arthritic patients. Phys Ther 64(4):504–509, 1984.
9. Winter, DA, et al: Kinematics of normal locomotion: A statistical study based on TV data. J Biomech 7(6):479–486, 1974.
10. Grundy, M, Tosh, PA, McLeish, RD, and Smidt, L: An investigation of the centers of pressure under the foot while walking. J Bone Joint Surg 57B(1):98–103, 1975.
11. Barnett, CH: The phases of human gait. Lancet 82(9)22:617–621, 1956.
12. Collis, WJ, and Jayson, MI: Measurement of pedal pressure. Ann Rheum Dis 31:215–217, 1972.
13. Scranton, PE, and McMaster, JH: Momentary distribution of forces under the foot. J Biomech 9:45–48, 1976.
14. Soames, RW: Foot pressure patterns during gait. J Biomed Eng 7(2):120–126, 1985.
15. Stokes, IAF, Stott, JRR, and Hutton, WC: Force distributions under the foot: A dynamic measuring system. Biomed Eng 9(4):140–143, 1974.
16. Cavanaugh, PR, and Michiyoshi, AC: A technique for the display of pressure distributions beneath the foot. J Biomech 13:69–75, 1980.
17. Grieve, DW, and Rashid, T: Pressure under normal feet in standing and walking as measured by foil pedobarography. Ann Rheum Dis 43:816–818, 1984.

# CHAPTER 3

# The Examination of the Foot

The foot and ankle are two of the segments of the human body, certainly of the neuromusculoskeletal system, that lend themselves to a complete "clinical" examination. The foot and ankle are readily accessible to visual, manual, palpatory, and functional evaluation.[1-3]

Pain and difficulty in walking are the usual symptoms that bring the patient to the physician. The patient literally "points" to the site of pain in the foot and ankle and indicates the manner in which there is dysfunction. The symptoms are either *static*, that is, pain or impairment during standing, or *kinetic*, that is, pain or impairment during walking, jumping, or running. The examination must be a systematic procedure to determine the precise deviation from normal.

The *normal foot* must conform to the following criteria: (1) must be pain free, (2) must exhibit normal muscle balance, (3) must have an absence of contracture, (4) must have a central heel, (5) must have straight and mobile toes, and (6) must have three sites of weight bearing during standing and during the stance phase of walking.

## HISTORY

The symptoms are subjective and revealed by the patient's history, which must be carefully and specifically guided. The site of pain and/or discomfort must be elicited and pointed out by the patient. The precise time (moment) of pain must be ascertained. The movement (kinetic) that (re)produces the pain must be determined, both in function and in specific foot-ankle movements. The site of pain indicated by the patient must be reproduced by the examiner to determine the precise anatomic site of pain production.

The gait, which has been discussed, must be witnessed by the examiner and be evaluated as to which functional aspect of the neuromusculoskeletal component of the foot-ankle is responsible. The examination must be orthopedic and neurologic. The history must reveal the probable cause considered responsible for the pain and impairment.

The footwear must be evaluated as indicating where there are abnormalities that have been caused by the abnormal gait or stance (Fig. 3–1). In the normal foot, the shoe becomes worn at the heel on its outer side at proper heel strike and with a proper dorsiflexion in inversion and the calcaneus centrally placed. An everted foot distorts the counter as the foot moves within its contour and causes deformity. Excessive wear of the toe of the shoe indicates inadequate dorsiflexion during the swing gait phase. Deformity of the vamp (upper part of shoe) may indicate abnormal toe flexion-extension and anatomic deformities of the toes.

Examination of the sole (Fig. 3–2) depicts the weight bearing of the foot (shoe) during gait as well as indicating the location of the metatarsal heads.

## CLINICAL EXAMINATION

Clinical examination must evaluate any or all of the tissue sites that may be the site and source of pain as well as the site and source of impairment. Every joint must be specifically evaluated, as must every tendon, ligament, nerve, and blood vessel. As stated, *all* are available to the examiner's eyes and fingers.

### Ankle

The ankle joint must be examined with the foot bare. The range of motion tested is essentially the talus within the mortise, which must be judged from the

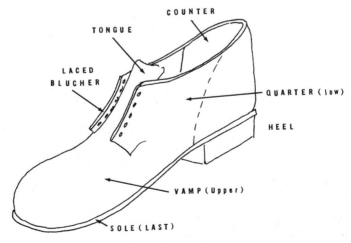

**Figure 3–1.** Components of the shoe. The standard components of a typical shoe are indicated.

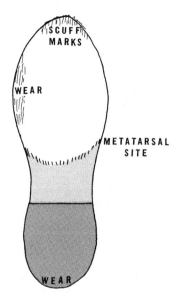

**Figure 3–2.** Examination of the sole of the shoe. Examination of the sole of a shoe indicates the sites of weight bearing during the stance phase, toe-off, and heel strike.

excursion of the hind foot rather than the forefoot since the forefoot's plantar flexion and dorsiflexion motions do not occur within the ankle mortise (Fig. 3–3).

Because testing the range of motion of the ankle also tests the flexibility of the gastrocnemius-soleus muscle group as well as the integrity of the joints, the

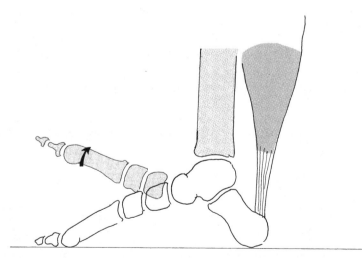

**Figure 3–3.** False impression of ankle dorsiflexion. The motion of the calcaneus indicates the range of motion of the foot-ankle complex. Dorsiflexion of the forefoot at the subtalar joint without calcaneal motion or elongation of the gastrocnemius-soleus group may give a false impression of range of motion.

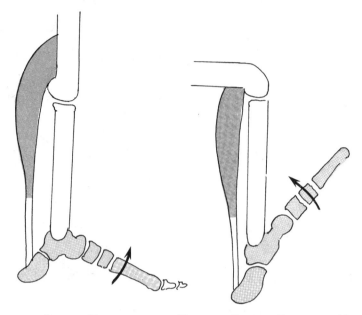

**Figure 3–4.** Influence of knee in testing ankle range of motion. In testing ankle plantar and dorsal flexion, the knee position must be considered as the gastrocnemius muscle originates above the knee joint. The gastrocnemius muscle will limit ankle dorsiflexion when the knee is extended as it will do so to a lesser degree with the knee flexed.

position of the knee during the examination must be ascertained. The gastrocnemius muscle originates above the knee joint and thus changes when the knee is extended or flexed. The soleus muscle attaches at the lower leg and thus is not associated with flexion of the knee (Fig. 3–4).

Figures 3–5 and 3–6 show the techniques of manually examining ankle range of motion. The foot and ankle move in dorsiflexion and plantar flexion and literally have no significant measurable translation motion since this action is limited by ligaments. During examination of the ankle, this motion must be tested, especially if ankle ligamentous pathology is considered (Fig. 3–7).

## Subtalar Joint

The subtalar and transverse tarsal joints work together, combining the movements of *inversion* and *eversion* (Figs. 3–8 and 3–9). Clinically it is possible to differentiate which joint is involved.

Subtalar motion is tested by holding the lower leg firmly with one hand and holding the calcaneus in the other while keeping the ankle dorsiflexed. In the dorsiflexed ankle position, the talus is firmly placed within the mortise, which

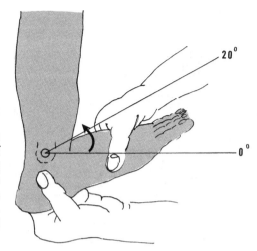

**Figure 3–5.** Ankle dorsiflexion: Range of motion. Dorsiflexion of the foot measuring the talus moving in the ankle mortise is tested by the examiner's left hand holding the calcaneus and the right hand passively dorsiflexing the foot. Normal range is usually to 20°.

prevents lateral and medial motion. Passive range of motion of the talocalcaneal joint is approximately 20° (Fig. 3–10).

## Metatarsal Joints

Motion of the forefoot at the metatarsal cuneiform-cuboid joints can also be tested. These articulations form the posterior metatarsal arch (Figs. 3–11 and 3–12). Midtarsal movement is tested by holding the heel firmly with one

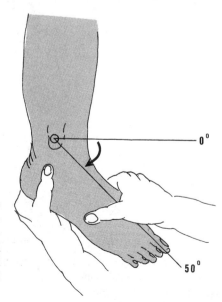

**Figure 3–6.** Ankle plantar flexion: Range of motion. Plantar flexion of the foot measuring the talus moving in the ankle mortise is tested by the examiner's left hand holding the calcaneus and the right hand passively plantarflexing the foot. Normal range is usually to 50°.

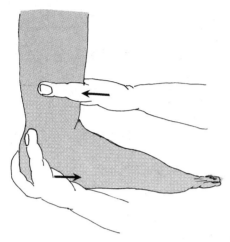

**Figure 3–7.** Ankle joint translation: Range of motion. Passive translation of the foot within the ankle mortise is usually very limited because the anterior talofibular ligament resists motion. The lower leg is resisted by the examiner's right hand, and the left hand cups the heel and pulls it forward. In a severe ligamentous injury such as strain, sprain, or tear (see text), there is excessive motion as compared to that in the opposite foot-ankle. This is known as an "anterior drawer sign."

hand and grasping the forefoot at the base of the metatarsals with the other hand. The examining hand pronates, supinates (Fig. 3–13), adducts, and abducts the forefoot (Fig. 3–14). Supination is greater than is pronation, a total of which is approximately 40°.

Testing the motion at the base of each metatarsal as it articulates with the cuneiforms and cuboid must be done individually since each articulation is dif-

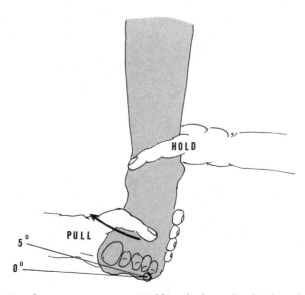

**Figure 3–8.** Forefoot inversion testing. Holding the lower leg firmly and grasping the forefoot using a medial motion with the examining hand to evaluate forefoot inversion (approximately 5°).

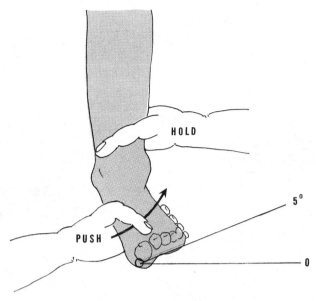

**Figure 3–9.** Forefoot eversion testing. Holding the lower leg firmly and grasping the forefoot using a lateral motion with the examining hand to evaluate forefoot eversion (approximately 5°).

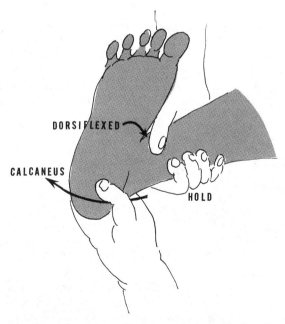

**Figure 3–10.** Talocalcaneal motion evaluation. With the ankle dorsiflexed, the anterior portion of the talus fits snuggly in the ankle mortise, allowing no lateral-medial motion. Mobilizing the calcaneus with the examining hand checks the motion of the talocalcaneal joint (approximately 20°).

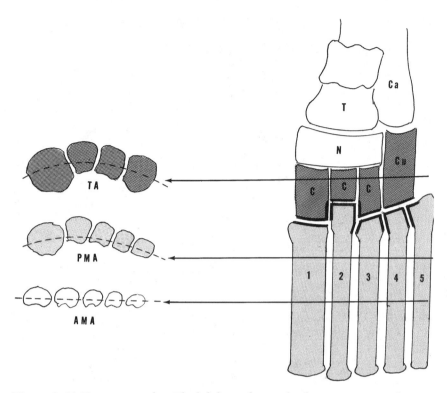

**Figure 3–11.** Transverse arches. The left figure depicts the three transverse arches: TA = tarsal arch; PMA = posterior metatarsal arch; and AMA = anterior metatarsal arch. The right figure shows the articulations of metatarsals 1, 2, 3, 4, and 5 with the tarsal row, the cuneiforms (C), and the cuboid (Cu). The darkened edges show the articulating surfaces. Metatarsal 2 base is in the mortise formed by the inner and outer cuneiforms and the shorter middle cuneiform. The tarsals include the cuboid (Cu), and the hindfoot includes the talus (T) and the calcaneus (Ca).

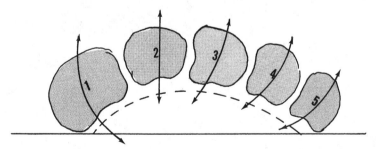

**Figure 3–12.** Transverse arch. Otherwise known as the posterior metatarsal arch, the transverse arch is formed by the base of the five metatarsals and is relatively fixed, although there is motion of each bone. The base of the second metatarsal (2) is wedged into the mortise formed by the medial and lateral cuneiforms and allows motion in only one plane: flexion and extension and with limited range. The first metatarsal (1) arcs about the base of the second metatarsal, and the third (3), fourth (4), and fifth (5) arc about their adjacent metatarsals in the opposite direction. Total flexion causes this arc to form a "cupping" of the base.

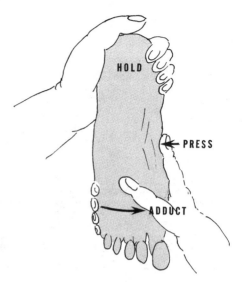

**Figure 3–13.** Forefoot adduction testing. Forefoot inversion is evaluated by holding calcaneus firmly and grasping the forefoot with the examining hand. Using a medial motion, the examining index finger is pressed against the navicular. The hand virtually holds the metatarsals and tests motion at their bases by articulating against the cuneiforms in both adduction-abduction and supination-pronation.

ferent. The technique of examination is similar (Fig. 3–15). It is only the expected motion that differs.

The first metarsal base is kidney-shaped, allowing plantar flexion and dorsiflexion to occur about an arc about the base. This allows "cupping" of the base, forming the transverse arch (see Fig. 3–12).

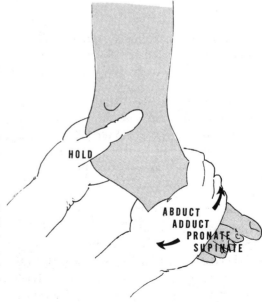

**Figure 3–14.** Testing motion at the midtarsal joints. By holding the hind foot firmly, the examining hand pronates, supinates, adducts, and abducts the forefoot, testing the metatarsaltarsal joints.

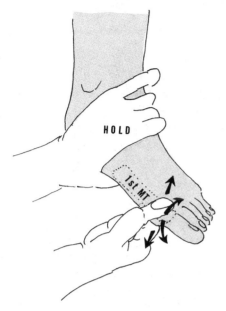

HOLD

1st MT

**Figure 3–15.** Examination of the first metatarsal-cuneiform articulation. The holding hand stabilizes the midtarsal bones, and the examining hand "pinches" the metatarsal (MT) being examined between the thumb and index finger. Each metatarsal is mobilized according to its normal motion (see accompanying text). In this illustration, the first metatarsal moves in dorsiplantar flexion (straight arrows) and in a circumferential motion as dictated by the shape of its base. As the examining fingers move laterally, each metatarsal is examined.

The base of the second metatarsal is square, fitting into a mortise formed by the three cuneiforms. This allows only plantar flexion and dorsiflexion (see Fig. 3–12) of that metatarsal.

The third, fourth, and fifth metatarsals move in a plantar and dorsal direction in a rotatory manner counter to the rotation of the first metatarsal. The fifth metatarsal contacts only the base of the fourth metatarsal, and the lateral aspect of the cuboid moves through the greatest arc. Metatarsal motion is essentially an arcuate movement in plantar flexion and dorsiflexion, the second metatarsal being fixed and the other moving in an arc about it, forming a flexible arc.

The metatarsophalangeal joints move in a specific direction and to a specific extent, depending on which toe is being evaluated and the fact that there are two phalanges in the first toe and three in the other four.

Because it is vitally involved in normal gait, the first ("big") toe must have an adequate range of motion to allow normal, pain-free motion. Range should approach 90° of dorsiflexion, with a range of only 60° being absolutely abnormal. Some abduction-adduction and rotation (Fig. 3–16) are passively possible, but not actively so.

## Ankle Ligaments

Ligaments that restrict joint range of motion are necessary for normal joint function. They are subject to examination visually by palpation and by passive and active joint motion. Their function and attachments are discussed in Chapter 1.

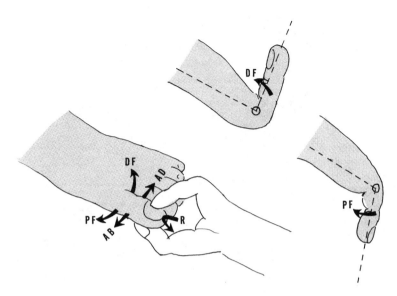

**Figure 3–16.** Examination of the hallux: Passive motion. Grasping the big toe between the index finger and thumb, the following motions can be elicited: Dorsiflexion (DF), normally 90°, and plantar flexion (PF), also 90°. Passively testing for abduction (AB) and adduction (AD) as well as rotation (R) indicates the integrity of the cartilage and possible deterioration.

The *deltoid ligament*, also called the medial collateral ligaments, is palpable just inferior to the medial malleolus and is directly palpable. Its integrity is tested by everting the hind foot (Fig. 3–17) and equating it with a similar motion of the other ankle.

There are three lateral collateral ligaments: the anterior talofibular, calcaneofibular, and posterior talofibular (Fig. 3–18). Their origin and attachments are obvious from their names. None of these ligaments is as broad or as strong as the medial (deltoid) ligament, nor are they specifically palpable. Their stabilizing function, however, can be readily palpable by inverting the foot and ankle (see Fig. 3–9) and performing the translation test (see Fig. 3–7).

The anterior talofibular ligament, which runs from the anterior portion of the lateral malleolus to the lateral aspect of the talar neck, is directly palpable by palpating the sinus tarsi (Fig. 3–19), which is just anterior to the lateral malleolus. The sinus tarsi is a depression filled by the extensor digitorum brevis muscle and a small pad of fat. By inverting the foot, the examining finger can palpate the lateral neck of the talus. Deep within the sinus is the calcaneotalar ligament, which cannot be directly palpated.

The calcaneofibular ligament stretches in a plantar direction from the lateral malleolus to insert into the lateral wall of the calcaneus. It may be torn, but usually only if there has also been a tear of the anterior talofibular ligament.

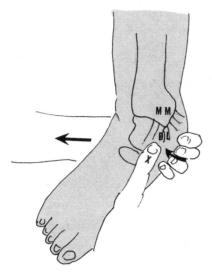

**Figure 3–17.** Palpating the deltoid ligament. During examination of the right foot, the medial malleolus (MM) is palpable. The examiner grasps the heel and everts it (curved arrow), putting the deltoid ligament (DL) under stress. Excessive passive motion can be determined by comparing the other ankle. The ligament can be palpated using the examining finger (X) of the other hand.

The posterior talofibular ligament originates from the posterior edge of the lateral malleolus and passes posteriorly to the small lateral tubercle on the posterior aspect of the talus. It is stronger than the other two lateral collateral ligaments and essentially prevents forward slippage of the fibula on the talus.

## Tendons

In examining the numerous joints of the foot and ankle to ascertain their normal flexibility, the tendons responsible for kinetic function must also be evaluated. Tendons may be visually observed as well as manually evaluated. Their function is also actively discernible.

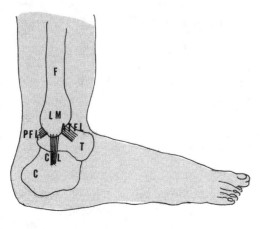

**Figure 3–18.** Lateral collateral ligaments of the ankle. The lateral collateral ligaments originate from the lateral malleolus (LM) at the distal end of the fibula (F). They are three in number: anterior talofibular (ATFL), attaching to the talus (T); the calcaneofibular (CFL), attaching to the calcaneus (C); and the posterior talofibular (PFL). They can be directly palpated, especially if the foot-ankle is passively inverted.

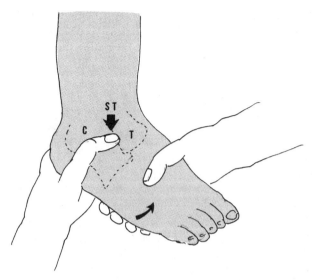

**Figure 3–19.** Palpation of the sinus tarsi. The sinus tarsi (ST) is a depression below the lateral malleolus between the talus (T) and the calcaneus (C). It can be palpated by slightly inverting the foot and palpating that depression. The talocalcaneal ligament is located within the sinus.

The *posterior tibialis tendon* is most prominent when the patient inverts and plantar flexes the foot. It is visible and palpable where it passes behind and inferior to the medial malleolus as the patient plantar flexes and inverts his or her foot (Fig. 3–20).

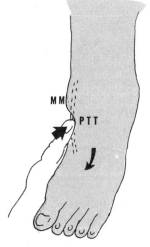

**Figure 3–20.** Palpation of the posterior tibialis tendon. The posterior tibialis tendon (PTT) is located immediately behind and under the medial malleolus (MM) and is directly palpable when the foot plantar flexes in an inverted direction (curved arrow).

The *flexor digitorum longus tendon* lies just behind the tibialis posterior tendon (see Fig. 3–21) and can be palpated while resisting the patient who flexes the toes while also plantar flexing and inverting the forefoot. The *flexor hallucis longus tendon* cannot be palpated because it lies on the posterior aspect of the ankle joint, deep to the muscles.

The *anterior tibialis tendon* is readily visible as the patient actively dorsiflexes and inverts the foot. It inserts onto the medial aspect of the base of the first metatarsal and first cuneiform bone (Fig. 3–21).

The *peroneus longus* and *peroneus brevis* tendons pass immediately behind the lateral malleolus (Fig. 3–22) as they cross the ankle joint. They evert and plantar flex the foot. They may be palpated at that site as the patient actively everts and plantar flexes the foot. As these tendons pass the calcaneus, they pass by the peroneal tubercle, which forms a "tunnel" between it and the lateral malleolus. The tendon ultimately inserts into the styloid process of the fifth metatarsal (Fig. 3–23). In palpating the styloid process, not only the peroneus tendon can be palpated but also by manually moving the process, the fifth metatarsocuboid joint can be tested.

The *hallucis longus muscle* (tendon) can be tested by resisting extension of the big toe and palpating the tendon (Fig. 3–24). Similarly, the outer four toe extensors can be tested by resisting their extension, thus testing the extensor digitorum longus and brevis (Fig. 3–25).

Toe flexors can also be manually tested (Fig. 3–26), and the small muscles of the foot served by the plantar nerves can be tested by "cupping" the foot (Fig. 3–27).

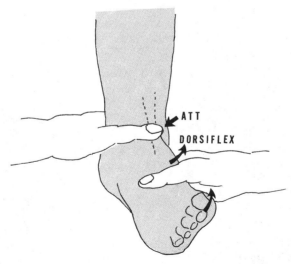

**Figure 3–21.** Palpation of the anterior tibialis tendon. As the foot actively dorsiflexes against the examiner's resistance, the anterior tibialis tendon (ATT) can be directly seen and palpated.

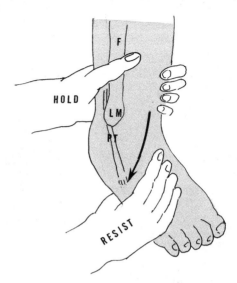

**Figure 3–22.** Testing peroneal function. The peroneal longus and brevis tendons (PT) pass behind the lateral malleolus (LM) at the distal end of the fibula (F) to attach to the styloid process. Its action is to plantar flex and evert the foot (curved arrow) and is tested by resisting that action.

## CIRCULATION

Blood is supplied to the foot and ankle by means of a continuation of the popliteal artery, which divides into the anterior tibial and the posterior tibial arteries. The popliteal artery is a direct continuation of the femoral artery, which passes into the posterior popliteal quadrant, where it divides (Fig. 3–28) into the posterior tibial and anterior tibial arteries.

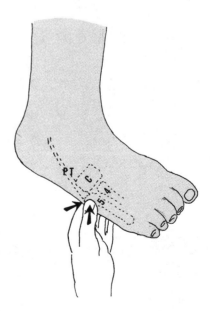

**Figure 3–23.** Palpation of the styloid process and the insertion of the peroneal tendons. The styloid process is palpable at the base of the fifth metatarsal (5). This is where the peroneal tendons (PT) insert. By moving the styloid process (arrows), the fifth metatarsal-cuboid (C) joint can be tested.

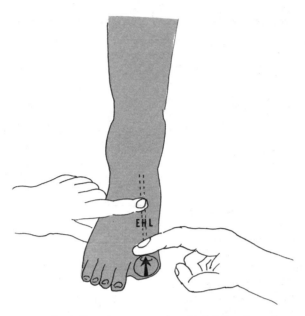

**Figure 3–24.** Testing the hallucis longus muscle. The left hand is palpating the hallucis longus tendon and the right hand resisting extension of the hallux. This muscle is innervated by the deep peroneal nerve with roots of L5, S1, and S2. The other toe extensors (examination not shown) require the resistance to be applied by the left hand over the outer four toes. This action is supplied by the extensor digitorum brevis with roots S1 and S2.

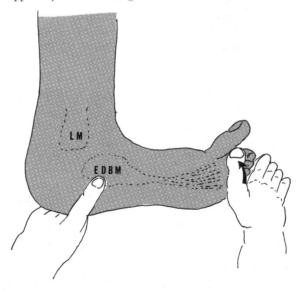

**Figure 3–25.** Testing extensor digitorum longus and brevis. The right hand is resisting extension of all the toes lateral to the hallux. The belly of the extensor digitorum brevis muscle (EDBM) (roots S1 and S2) can be palpated just below and ahead of the lateral malleolus (LM) and here is palpated by the left-hand index finger. The extensor digitorum longus muscle (roots L5, S1, and S2) is not shown.

84

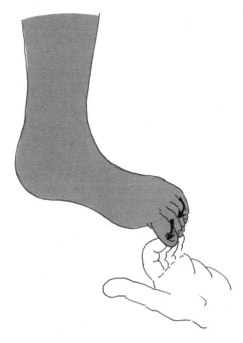

**Figure 3–26.** Manual testing of the toe flexors other than the hallux. Active flexion of all the toes (curved arrows) other than the hallux can be tested as shown.

The posterior tibial artery follows the same path as the tibial nerve, coursing around and behind the medial malleolus of the ankle (Fig. 3–29), supplying the posterior muscles of the leg until it divides at the plantar surface of the foot into the *medial* and *lateral* plantar arteries. Because they are too small and too deep, these are not directly palpable.

Below the popliteal quadrant, the popliteal artery bifurcates, forming the *anterior tibial artery*, which passes anteriorly between the tibia and the fibula

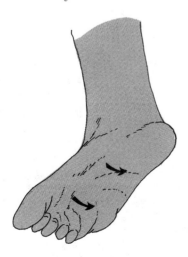

**Figure 3–27.** "Cupping" the sole of the foot. "Cupping" of the foot is possible by using the action of the small muscles of the foot. These muscles are supplied by the medial and lateral plantar nerves, which are branches of the posterior tibial nerve on the plantar surface of the foot. This illustration is a view of the foot looking at the sole.

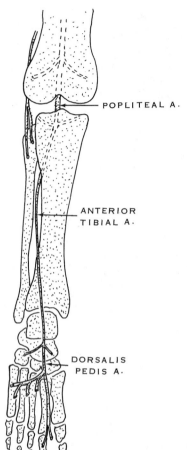

POPLITEAL A.

ANTERIOR
TIBIAL A.

DORSALIS
PEDIS A.

**Figure 3–28.** Arterial supply to the lower extremity.

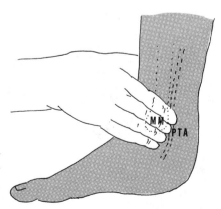

M M
PTA

**Figure 3–29.** Palpation of the posterior tibial artery. The posterior tibial artery (PTA) can be palpated just behind and curving under the medial malleolus (MM).

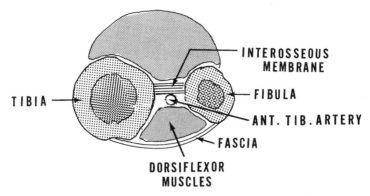

**Figure 3–30.** Interosseous membrane. Dorsal view of the interosseous membrane that connects the tibia and fibula. The anterior tibial artery (Ant. Tib. Artery) descends along the anterior border of the membrane. The fascia forms the anterior wall of the anterior compartment containing the dorsiflexor muscles.

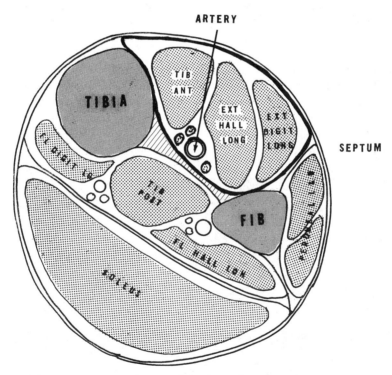

**Figure 3–31.** Anterior compartment of the lower leg. The anterior compartment is located within a fibrous sheath in the anterior portion of the lower leg. Posteriorly there is a firm, fibrous septum between the tibia and the fibula. Within the compartment is located the tibial artery and veins and the anterior tibial, extensor hallucis longus, and extensor digitorum longus muscles. Trauma to, or compression of, this compartment results in edema, which because it is firmly enclosed within the septa, leads to atrophy of the enclosed muscles and the nerves. The end result is termed an *anterior compression syndrome*.

through an opening in the superior aspect of the interosseous membrane, which connects the two bones and proceeds down the anterior surface of the membrane. During its passage, the anterior tibial artery supplies the muscles of the anterior compartment of the leg (Figs. 3–30 and 3–31).

As the anterior tibial artery reaches the dorsum of the foot, it becomes the dorsalis pedis artery (Fig. 3–32), the terminal branches of which form the *dorsal metatarsal arteries* and *dorsal digital arteries*. These communicate with the plantar distal branches of the plantar arteries.

Below the bifurcation of the popliteal artery, the artery branches off laterally, passes across the interosseous membrane, and descends the lateral aspect of the leg, supplying the lateral muscles of the leg. It ends as the *lateral calcaneal artery*.

The status of the circulation of the foot is determined by the presence or absence of edema, dependent cyanosis, warmth or coldness of the skin, dryness or moistness of the skin, and blanching of the elevated foot and leg.

When there is a suspicion of impaired circulation, either by objective evaluation or by subjective symptoms, palpation of arterial pulsations is the most significant test available to the clinician. Pain in the form of claudication is the most frequent symptom that alerts the patient to impaired circulation.

The dorsalis pedis artery and the posterior tibial artery are those most frequently palpated clinically. Many diagnostic procedures, such as Doppler testing and angiography, are now available that can accurately determine the status of circulation. These procedures can be used by a specialist when impaired circulation has been suspected and/or ascertained by the primary physician.

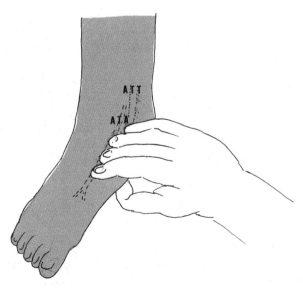

**Figure 3–32.** Palpation of the anterior tibial artery. The anterior tibial artery (ATA) descends along the dorsum of the foot lateral to the anterior tibial tendon (ATT).

## NEUROLOGIC EVALUATION

The lower extremity, and thus the foot, is innervated by branches of the sciatic nerve (L4, L5, S1, S2, and S3). Above the knee, as the sciatic nerve passes into the popliteal fossa, it divides into the tibial and common peroneal nerves.[4]

The *tibial nerve*, which is a continuation of the sciatic nerve, enters the lower leg between the two heads of the gastrocnemius muscle and then passes deep to the soleus muscle to enter the posterior compartment of the leg (Fig. 3–33).

The tibial nerve supplies the posterior muscles of the leg and innervates the plantar flexors of the foot. It terminates in medial and lateral divisions of the plantar nerves.

The *medial plantar nerve* (Fig. 3–34) sends cutaneous branches to the plantar surface of the medial three toes and the medial aspect of the fourth toe.

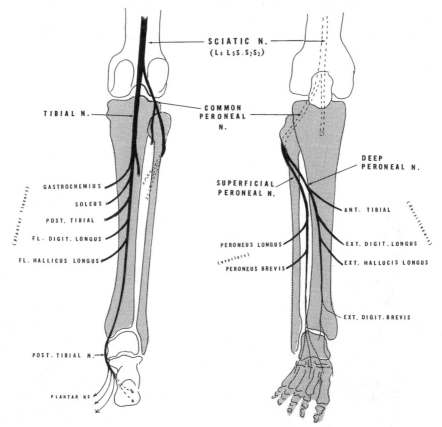

**Figure 3–33.** Innervation of the lower leg and foot.

Its motor branches supply the abductor hallucis, flexor digitorum brevis, and the first two lumbricales (Figs. 3–35, 3–36, 3–37, and 3–38).

The *lateral plantar nerve* passes across the plantar surface of the foot and ultimately divides into a deep and a superficial branch. It supplies sensation to the plantar surface of the foot (see Fig. 3–33). It also supplies the motor function to the quadratus plantae, flexor digiti quinti brevis, abductor digiti quinti, and the remaining plantar interosseous and lumbrical muscles.

The other division of the sciatic nerve, the *common peroneal nerve*, passes laterally out of the popliteal space. It passes behind the head of the fibula, beneath the deep fascia, and winds around the lateral aspect of the fibular neck. This nerve supplies *no* musculature. It supplies small twigs to the knee joint, and then divides into the superficial and deep peroneal nerves (see Fig. 3–32).

The *superficial peroneal nerve* descends the leg in front of the fibula and supplies the evertors of the foot. Its sensory branch supplies the lateral aspect of the lower leg and the dorsum of the foot (Fig. 3–39).

The *deep peroneal nerve* proceeds to the interosseous membrane between the fibula and tibia and descends the leg, supplying the extensor digitorum brevis. It supplies a small area of sensation between the two first toes on the dorsum of the foot. Both the deep and the superficial peroneal nerves terminate in sensory branches that supply the dorsum of the foot and the anterolateral aspect of the leg (see Fig. 3–39).

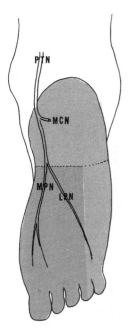

**Figure 3–34.** Dermatomal distribution of the plantar nerves. The posterior tibial nerve (PTN) divides into the medial plantar nerve (MPN) and the lateral plantar nerve (LPN). The dermatome area of the medial plantar nerve is the darker shade of the medial four toes. The lateral area (not delineated) of the anterior foot and outer toe and lateral aspect of toe 4 are supplied by the lateral plantar nerve. The heel area (within dotted line) is supplied by the medial calcaneal nerve (MCN), which branches from the posterior tibial nerve.

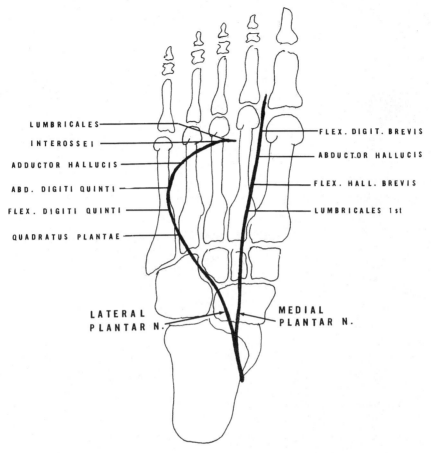

**Figure 3–35.** Muscles of the foot innervated by the plantar nerves.

## EVALUATION OF THE TIBIA-FIBULA AND FEMUR

Because the foot statically and kinetically is dependent on the ankle mortise, which in turn is dependent on the alignment of the tibia, the tibia, fibula, and femur all have to be evaluated.[5–7]

The tibial tuberosity should be directly under the patella, and in the flexed, dependent position of the lower leg, the dependent foot should *invert* slightly (Fig. 3–40). If there is aggravation of the inversion of the entire foot, an *internal tibial torsion* can be suspected. This is a rotation of the lower leg about the longitudinal axis. In the seated position with the lower leg dangling passively, the tibial tuberosity should be directly under the patella and the foot inverted slightly. In *external tibial torsion* the opposite situation is noted.

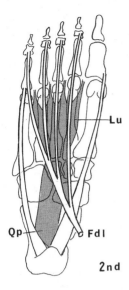

**Figure 3–36.** Muscles of the sole of the foot: second layer. Qp = quadratus plantae; Lu = lumbricales; Fdl = tendon of flexor digitorum longus.

In the standing position (Fig. 3–41), the torsion of the tibia on the femur or the femur on the tibia can be noted. These are conditions known as "pigeon-toed," "Charlie Chaplin gait," waddling, bow-legged, knock-kneed, and genu recurvatum. It behooves the examiner observing this gait or stance to fully evaluate the entire extremity and not merely the foot and ankle.[8–10]

With any of these conditions noted, the hip joint requires evaluation. In alteration of the *angle of anteversion* (Fig. 3–42), the angle of the femoral neck

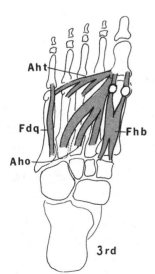

**Figure 3–37.** Muscles of the sole of the foot: third layer. Aht = adductor hallucis: transverse head; Aho = adductor hallucis: oblique head; Fhb = flexor hallucis brevis; Fdq = flexor digiti quinti brevis.

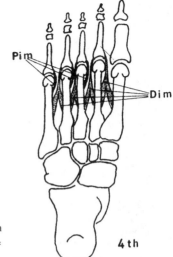

**Figure 3–38.** Muscles of the sole of the foot: fourth layer. Pim = plantar interosseous muscles; Dim = dorsal interosseous muscles.

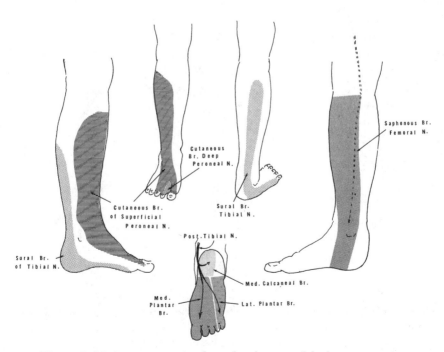

**Figure 3–39.** Sensory patterns of peripheral nerves of the lower extremity.

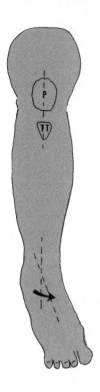

**Figure 3–40.** Normal tibial torsion. In viewing the seated person (here the right leg), a line drawn through the patella (P) and the tibial tubercle (TT) is transected by a line drawn through the foot. Normally there is a slight internal rotation, as indicated here.

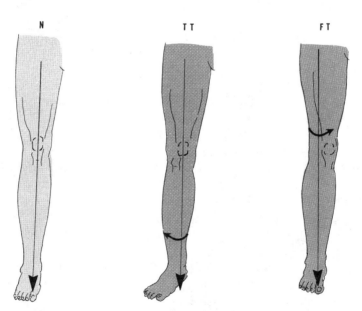

**Figure 3–41.** Torsions of lower extremity. N is the normal alignment in which the plumb line transects the patella and touches the foot between the first and second toe. TT (tibial torsion) depicts external rotation of the tibia upon the femur, and FT, femoral torsion of the femur upon the tibia (curved arrows).

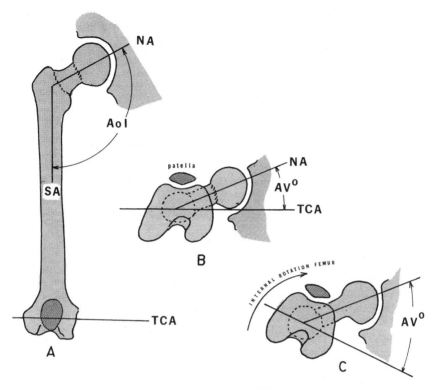

**Figure 3–42.** Angle of anteversion. The transcondylar axis (TCA) is a transverse line passing through the femoral condyles. An axis placed through the femoral neck (NA) forms an angle with TCA, which is called the *angle of anteversion*. This is angle AV° in part *B* with the femoral head viewed from above. A 15 to 25° angle is considered normal. In *C*, the angle is increased due to internal rotation of the femur in relationship to the femoral neck. This is increased anteversion. Viewing the femur from anterior-posterior direction, *A* depicts the *angle of inclination* (see Fig. 3-43). SA = angle of shaft; AoI = angle of inversion.

as the head of the femur is seated in the acetabulum is determined. The transcondylar axis represents a plane passing side by side through the femur. The normal range of anteversion is 15 to 25°. An increase in this angle is an increase in anteversion, which results in *internal femoral rotation*. This causes a gait termed *toeing in*.

The *angle of inclination* must also be determined (Fig. 3–43). This is the angle of the neck of the femoral head to the shaft of the femur. This angle is normally 116 to 140° with a greater angle forming *coxa valga* and a lesser angle *coxa vara*.

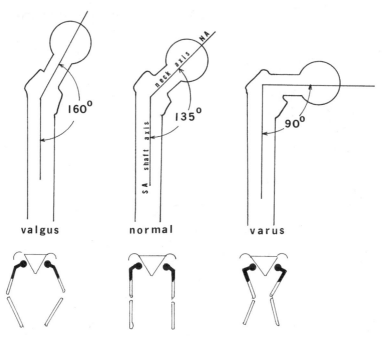

**Figure 3–43.** Angle of inclination. The angle formed by intersecting the femoral neck angle (NA) with an axis drawn through the shaft (SA) of the femur is termed the *angle of inclination*. This angle normally varies between 116 to 140° with the average being 135°.

## GENU

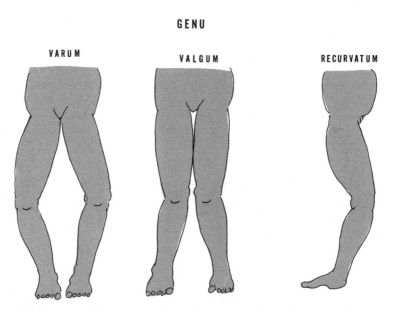

**Figure 3–44.** Knee deformities: *Left*, genu varum (bowlegged); *center*, genu valgum (knock-kneed); *right*, genu recurvatum (back-kneed). These are common deformities. They can impede or impair the gait and, when severe, can malalign the feet and ankles.

Another aspect of the foot and legs that requires observation as to their influence on gait is the angulation of the knee: *genu varum (bow-leg)*, *genu valgum (knock-knee)*, and *genu recurvatum (back knee)* (Fig. 3–44).

# REFERENCES

1. Basmajian, JV: Grant's Method of Anatomy, ed 8. Williams & Wilkins, Baltimore, 1971.
2. Cailliet, R: Foot and ankle pain, Chap. 13, in Soft Tissue Pain and Disability, ed 2. FA Davis, Philadelphia, 1996.
3. Fleming, LL (ed): Management of foot problems. Orthop Clin North Am 20:4, 1989.
4. Haymaker, W, and Woodhall, B: Peripheral Nerve Injuries: Principles of Diagnosis, ed 2. WB Saunders, Philadelphia, 1952.
5. Hollinshead, WH: Functional Anatomy of the Limbs and Back. WB Saunders, Philadelphia, 1952.
6. Inman, VT, Ralston, HJ, and Todd, F: Human Walking. Williams & Wilkins, Baltimore, 1981.
7. Root, M, Orien, WP, and Weed, JH: Normal and Abnormal Function of the Foot: Clinical Biomechanics, Vol 2. Clinical Biomechanics Corporation, Los Angeles, 1977.
8. Sussman, A, and Goode, R: The Magic of Walking. Simon & Schuster, New York, 1967.
9. Walther, D: Applied Kinesiology, Vol 1. SDC Systems DC, Pueblo, Colorado, 1981.
10. The Professional Staff Association: Observational Gait Analysis Handbook. Rancho Los Amigos Medical Center, Downey, California, 1989.

# CHAPTER 4

# The Foot in Childhood

If recognized and treated early, many foot problems commonly seen at birth and during early childhood may respond to appropriate conservative treatment and not lead to subsequent problems. Such abnormalities are more frequent than the literature indicates and possibly fail to be recognized because their mechanisms and ultimate development are not fully appreciated.

## CLASSIFICATION OF FOOT DEFORMITIES

Foot deformities are generally classified into four categories based on the position of the foot: (1) *equinus*, in which the heel is elevated and the foot plantar-flexed; (2) *calcaneus*, in which the foot is dorsiflexed and the heel relatively depressed; (3) *varus*, in which the foot is inverted and adducted; and (4) *valgus*, in which the foot assumes a position of eversion and abduction.

The terminology[1] here requires some clarification:

1. *Varus* implies that the distal member of an extremity is bent "toward" the midline. The apex of the angle formed by the longitudinal axes of the component bones points *away from* the midline. The heel is rotated inward on its longitudinal axis or is inverted.
2. *Valgus* means bent or turned "from" the midline. The apex formed by the longitudinal axes of the component bones points *toward* the midline. In valgus, the heel is everted or rotated outward on its longitudinal axis.
3. Position about an axis passing transversely through the foot is termed *dorsiflexion* or *plantar flexion*, whereas a position about a vertical axis is termed *abduction* or *adduction* and a position about a longitudinal axis is termed *inversion* or *eversion*. Inversion implies elevation of the inner

border of the foot, and eversion, elevation of the outer border. Adduction-abduction occurs chiefly at the tarsometatarsal joints. Inversion and adduction combine to constitute *supination* and *varus* of the forefoot. *Pronation* is eversion and abduction of the foot (Fig. 4–1).

MacConail[2] views the foot as a "twisted osteo fibrous plate" by which the intrauterine position of the child's foot is in pronation and by "untwisting" becomes supinated at birth or thereafter. Normal foot postures and deformities usually consist of any combination of positions, with equinus associated with varus or valgus and calcaneus with varus or valgus. This concept may be questioned as the fetal position is that of inversion and supination (Fig. 4–2), depending on the fetal age at which it is evaluated.

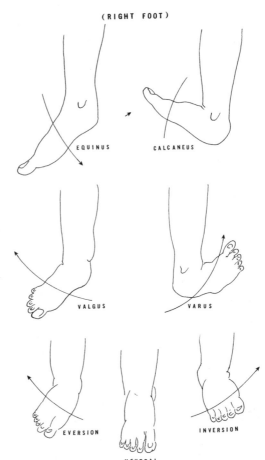

**Figure 4–1.** The terminology of abnormal foot positions.

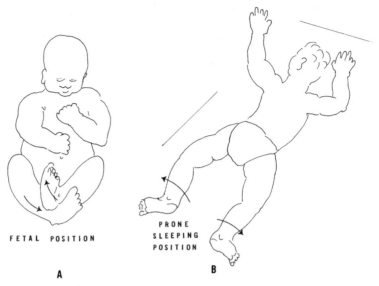

FETAL  POSITION

PRONE
SLEEPING
POSITION

A

B

**Figure 4–2.** Fetal and sleeping postures. *A* depicts the fetal position with the hips flexed, abducted, and outwardly rotated. The feet are usually plantar-flexed and adducted with their plantar surfaces against the abdomen. *B* is the sleeping position of the newborn with the thighs externally rotated and the feet abducted. These foot positions vary, depending on the intrauterine position prior to birth.

## ETIOLOGIC CONCEPTS

The majority of foot deformities noted in infants are flatfoot or equinovarus deformities with valgus, varus, equinus, and calcaneus abnormalities seen in a lesser percentage. Most of these abnormalities are considered to be either congenital, acquired, or a residue of a neurologic abnormality.

An intriguing concept is that of delayed or arrested derotation of the foot from the intrauterine position. At about the third month of intrauterine existence, the fetus's thighs are flexed, abducted, and outwardly rotated and the lower portions of its legs are crossed. The feet are plantar-flexed and adducted, with the plantar surfaces held against the fetal abdomen. As the fetus develops, the thighs derotate inwardly and the feet gradually turn outward, pressing against the uterine wall.

If, for any reason, there is an alteration or cessation of the rotational aspects of the feet, the child is born with the feet in that position. With regard to the congenital clubfoot (discussed later), in 1969 J. Leonard Goldner[3] stated "that much remains to be learned about the basic defect that causes the clubfoot deformity." Twenty some years later, this statement still remains valid.[4]

Newborns may have a postural attitude of one leg internally rotated and the other externally rotated. This is a condition termed *windblown hips*, the analogy being that of a sailor walking against the wind. Because the child may continue to sleep in this position, the tissues of the lower extremity will so adapt.

The tissues involved in a fetal and newborn position will adapt to that position. The soft tissues "contract" and the bones so deform, as do the articulations. At birth, the foot of the infant is as much soft tissue as it is bone. X-rays of the foot show only the diaphysis of the phalanges, the metatarsal, and the nuclei of the calcaneus and talus (Fig. 4–3).

As growth continues through adolescence, the foot undergoes ossification and fusion at varying ages (Fig. 4–4). By the time of adulthood, the foot is 90% bone.

## EXAMINATION OF THE NEWBORN FOOT

In a visually apparent deformity of the non-weight-bearing foot, manual testing will determine the deformity and whether there is sufficient flexibility for correction. Not only the foot but also the ankle, lower leg, femur, and hip joints must be examined. Treatment of the specific soft-tissue deformity must address these deformities by persistent stretching and also by possible casting. Each deformity will be addressed in this therapeutic regard. Overcorrection is often indicated because a slow partial return to the initial deforming soft tissue is to be expected.

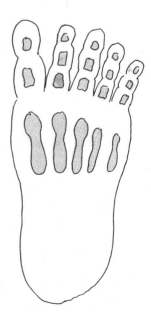

**Figure 4–3.** X–ray of newborn foot. In the newborn, only the diaphysis of the phalanges and the metatarsals are visible along with the nuclei of the talus and calcaneus.

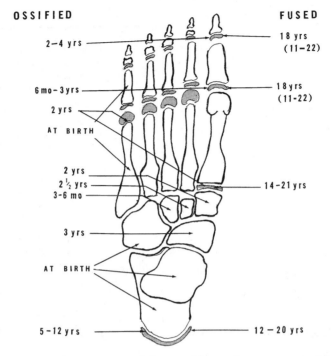

**Figure 4–4.** Age of appearance and closure of the ossification centers of the foot.

## THE PRONATED OR "FLAT" FOOT

The infant foot is and appears to be "flat." No longitudinal arch is noted because it is either not anatomically present or the arch is filled with a fat pad. The navicular and cuneiform that form the apex of the longitudinal arch are still in their cartilaginous stage and are soft and compressible. The muscles and ligaments are not yet well developed, and the foot is not yet ready for weight bearing. It has been considered that age 2 is the weight-bearing stage, yet earlier walking is possible and should be permitted.

Because a pronated foot is considered as "normal" in the infant, only a severe degree of pronation, which may concern parents, must be addressed. There are three degrees of pronation: (1) mild, or first degree; (2) moderate, or second degree, and (3) severe, or third degree. First degree places the weight-bearing line along medial border of the foot with some visible longitudinal arch. Second-degree changes the contour of the foot with depression of the longitudinal arch and prominence of the navicular bone. A third-degree pronation is a "totally flat foot" with no longitudinal arch and a footprint that reveals no indentation along the inner border. Because these gradations (degrees) are arbitrary, they do not influence the choice of treatment or indicate the ultimate severity of any symptoms that may evolve regarding the foot.

## Congenital Flatfoot

The true *congenital* flatfoot, (Fig. 4–5) is relatively rare, but when present, is more severe the "acquired" flatfoot. If the congenital flatfoot is flexible, the position of the calcaneovalgus is that of the foot folded laterally on itself. Being flexible, it can easily be manually corrected and thus maintained until adequate muscular action and weight bearing develop.

Therapeutically, manual correction of the forefoot is by means of daily exercises and by fitting with a custom-molded shoe that holds the foot in the corrected position. A bivalved plaster cast molding of the foot in the desired position may be applied for correction and then used occasionally during development for more minor correction not accomplished by exercise or the shoe.

## Rigid Flatfoot

The *rigid*, inflexible flatfoot is more difficult to treat. In this condition, the heel is firmly held in a marked valgus position and the forefoot in marked eversion. There is almost a reversal of the longitudinal arch, which appears to be convex rather than concave with bulging at the midpoint. X-rays reveal the talus

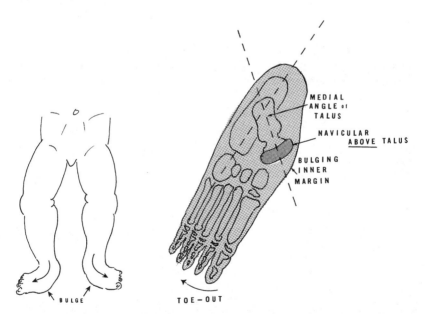

**Figure 4–5.** Congenital flatfoot. This is a calcaneovalgus foot. The heel is in valgus, and the talus points medially toward the other foot, forming an angle with the calcaneus. The talus points downward rather than forward, and the navicular lies on the superior surface of the neck of the talus instead of anterior to the head.

facing medially and downward and the navicular resting on the superior surface of the neck of the talus rather than in front of the head.

Correction of this condition requires a series of corrective plaster casts that change the convexity of the longitudinal arch and return the navicular to its normal position ahead of the head of the talus. The former is relatively easy, but the latter may require surgical intervention.

The result may be disappointing with surgical arthrodesis being required in later life if the gait is abnormal and painful.

## Acquired Flatfoot

The *acquired* flatfoot is usually flexible and may appear well formed when not weight bearing but on weight bearing assumes a flattened position. The longitudinal arch that appeared normal on non–weight bearing now is effaced, and the medial border of the foot loses its concavity and appears to bulge as the navicular is depressed toward the floor. The calcaneus undergoes eversion. It is interesting that arising up on the toes much of the longitudinal arch is regained only to be lost upon weight bearing.

Children with acquired flatfoot have an awkward gait. They walk with a "toe-out gait" and lack "spring" in their heel off phase. They often complain of calf ache. These complaints to parents are the usual cause that brings them to their physician.

Many acquired flatfoot patients also have generalized ligamentous laxity, which is noted in the hips, knees, elbows, low back, and even the upper extremities. These children are known as "double jointed" as an expression of their excessive flexibility.

Hypoflexibility, in which there is limited extensibility of the gastrocnemius-soleus–Achilles tendon complex causing pronation during stance and gait, may cause pronation of the foot. The limited ankle dorsiflexion is noted during a careful manual examination.

## Internal Tibial Torsion

Severe *internal tibial torsion* causing an inverted foot stance and gait, a "toe-in gait," may be compensated for by intentional "toe-out" gait, which causes the foot to pronate and should be evaluated.

Internal tibial torsion of a significant degree rarely persists after infancy. It has been estimated that 10% of children reaching the age of 5 have significant residual internal tibial torsion with less than 5% persisting into adolescence. Because this is an accepted fact, treatment of internal tibial torsion is rarely indicated.

Pronation may be acquired after prolonged bed rest or after prolonged immobilization of the foot and leg in a plaster cast for any condition. It has been assumed that internal tibial torsion is acquired from faulty sleeping habits during the first 4 months of life, during which the child sleeps in a "frog position" (see *B* in Fig. 4–2), in which the child lies prone with hips flexed, abducted, and externally rotated. A very firm mattress and bulky diapers encourage this posture. The pressure on the medial aspect of the foot in this lower-extremity position allegedly causes pronation by stretching the invertors and allowing the evertors to become contracted.

The usual normal sitting posture of a child—with the hips externally rotated and the feet under the child—is acceptable unless this position is prolonged and during this seated posture the feet are turned outward, causing the floor pressure to be against the inner border of the foot, causing pronation.

## Treatment of the Pronated Foot

The pronated foot must be treated before the child becomes ambulatory. Prewalking treatment consists in altering the observed sleeping pattern, gaining and maintaining flexibility of the entire lower extremity. The noted internal rotation of the lower extremity must be addressed with daily stretching. The foot must be exercised to acquire a longitudinal arch and a supinated foot. Exercises, which must be done daily and correctly, must be clearly outlined and demonstrated to the parents.

Proper use of pillows can avoid faulty sleeping postures. This requires looking at the child frequently during his or her sleep or during napping. Multiple, thick diapers must be avoided.

If there is limitation of flexibility of the hips, during either external or internal rotation, then the hip must be frequently stretched by means of passive exercise during the day. This is done by placing the child in the supine position with the legs extended, and then flexed to 90° and gently but firmly externally (or internally) rotating the upper legs to their limits and holding them for several seconds each episode. The parent is instructed to *gently but firmly* "stretch the tissues to their limits."

The foot (feet) must be manually stretched into adduction and supination frequently and then held in the newly acquired position for 30 to 40 seconds. The manual technique of stretching is shown in Fig. 4–6, which depicts an adult foot; however, the technique is the same for a child, using different pressure sites since the foot is smaller.

Once ambulation begins, the toe-out gait and weight-bearing pronation can be noted. Gait and stance are awkward. The child stands with feet turned out and walks with little "spring" in the gait.

If the child has a significant internal tibial torsion, the gait is toe-in in spite of the foot being pronated. This gait causes the foot to supinate, thus forming a longitudinal arch. This should be encouraged, or at least not prevented, since the gait will ultimately modify and the foot remain supinated. These contradic-

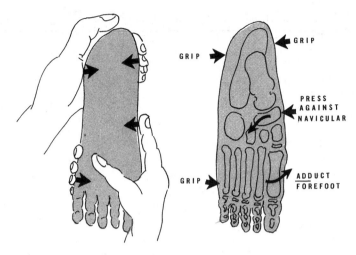

**Figure 4–6.** Manual correction of flatfoot deformity. Illustration demonstrates the technique of manually correcting the deformity of the right foot. The heel is gripped by the therapist's left hand, holding the calcaneus in a neutral position. The index finger of the right hand presses against the navicular bone as the other fingers move the forefoot in an adducted direction about the navicular axis. For the left foot the opposite is done.

tions require careful evaluation of the foot and the gait and determination as to which needs attention or which merely needs observation but no intervention.

The obese phlegmatic child is more prone to having pronated feet. Weight reduction should be undertaken and proper walking activity encouraged albeit in play activities.

## Shoe Corrections (Orthosis)

In the newborn, no shoe corrections are indicated. However, when the deformity is significant, correction is done with exercise, plaster casts, or even orthotic appliances. A "shoe" applied can only maintain the correction otherwise gained.

In a normal child, shoes must merely fit the foot and protect against external obstacles. The shoe must be adequately wide to prevent constriction. A high-top shoe does not afford support and is only of cosmetic value.

The shoe for a child with deformity must specifically address that deformity. The last of the shoe must address the desired shape of the foot. In the pronated foot, the last must turn "in" and the heel must be held snuggly within the counter (Fig. 4–7). Any correction that does not control the heel is fraught with failure. Pronation can be partially and significantly corrected by inverting the heel with a snug counter and a medial heel-wedge insert of as little as 1/16

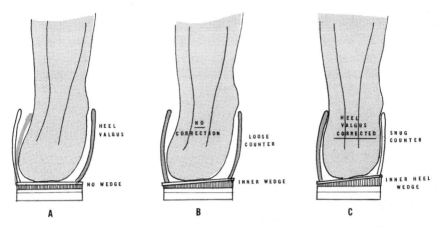

**Figure 4–7.** Necessity of a snug counter in shoe correction. *A* shows valgus of the heel within a normal shoe. An inner wedge insert (*B*) with a loose counter does *not* correct the valgus. A snug counter (*C*) and an insert has corrective value to heel valgus.

to 3/16 inch (Fig. 4–8). A Thomas heel (Fig. 4–9) is frequently prescribed. This type of heel has the advantage that, as the foot progresses forward during the stance phase, the anterior protrusion of the heel presents a site of internal rotation of the foot during that phase of stance.

The shank of the shoe should not be too firm and inflexible because this prevents the intrinsic muscles of the foot from functioning.

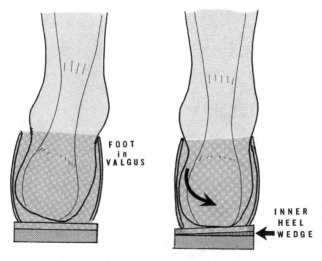

**Figure 4–8.** Inner wedge shoe insert. In treating a heel valgus, an inner wedge with a 1/16 to 3/16 inch elevation and the shoe counter being snug cause the foot to invert and supinate.

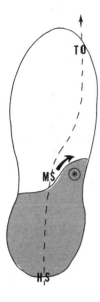

**Figure 4–9.** Thomas heel function. The foot stance during gait starts at heel strike (HS) and progresses through the midstance phase (MS), at which point the anterior ledge of the Thomas heel (°) becomes the site of internal rotation (arrow), causing supination of the foot as it progresses to toe-off (TO).

Arch supports are indicated in correcting and maintaining the corrected pronated foot. They allegedly maintain the longitudinal arch. Arch supports of whatever material should be molded over a plaster-casted foot of the patient molded into the desired posture of the foot. The orthosis affords pressure under the navicular with the forward portion extending behind the first three metatarsal heads and to the lateral aspect of the foot including the heel.

This type of orthosis may be made of felt or sponge-covered leather that has been molded. The leather orthosis is flexible and does deform on weight bearing but is elevated at the apex of the longitudinal arch. The orthosis may also be made of metal or plastic, which is less flexible and often causes pressure that is unacceptable to the patient. An orthosis that is uncomfortable will not be worn and thus will not be corrective.

The Biomechanics Laboratory of the University of California has designed an orthosis called the UC-BL Shoe Insert (Fig. 4–10). This orthosis is constructed from a plaster cast–molded foot of the patient, which has been covered with a skin-tight rubber on which is molded a fiberglass orthosis. When completed, this orthosis is a skin-tight corrective device that totally encloses the foot.

## Exercises: Gait Training

The most beneficial method of treating a pronated foot is exercise, because the musculature that forms the normal foot must be strengthened.

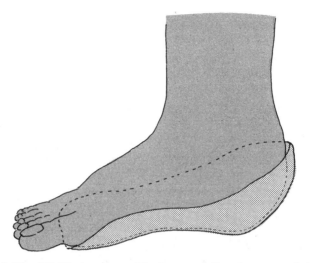

**Figure 4–10.** The UC-BL shoe insert. The laminated fiberglass insert shell is molded over a plaster mold of the foot. It fits snugly into the shoe. The heel is held in a neutral position, and the forefoot held in an adducted, supinated position.

Arch supports and corrective shoes are merely *passive* supports, whereas exercises are *active*. The age of child, the length of the attention span, and the ability to cooperate are obviously important in prescribing and performing exercises.

The heel cord–gastrocnemius-soleus complex must be sufficiently flexible to allow 90° of dorsiflexion. This can be accomplished passively. The gastrocnemius-soleus muscle group must be strong, and thus toe walking, or rising up on the toes, is a good exercise. The intrinsic muscles of the foot can be strengthened by picking up marbles with the toes or wrinkling a towel with the toes. Standing on the outer borders of the feet and simultaneously curling the toes strengthens these intrinsics.

Teaching walking with a heel-toe gait and the feet turned out about 10° from midline is a good gait-training process. In severe cases or in an uncooperative child, "twisters" (Fig. 4–11) may be used.

## METATARSUS VARUS

*Metatarsus varus* is a common condition in newborns (Fig. 4–12). This condition was originally termed adductus, and these terms remain identical and

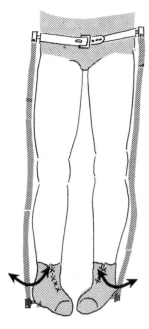

**Figure 4–11.** Orthotic "twisters" to control internal or external rotation. The "twisters" are coiled springs within a cable housing that resists torque. By means of its attachment at the pelvic band and to the shoe, the foot can be adjusted to turn "in" or "out" as the condition demands. This twister allows ambulation yet controlling the lower extremity in both the stance or swing phase of the gait cycle.

interchangeable. In this condition, the foot has an adducted forefoot, a convex lateral border, and the heel is in valgus.

The following components establish the proper diagnosis and ensure appropriate treatment (Fig. 4–13):

1. The anterior segment of the foot is in adduction.
2. The lateral border of the foot is convex.
3. The heel is in valgus.
4. Internal tibial torsion is frequently present.
5. There is a sharp angulation of the medial border of the foot at the metatarsal joint.
6. The first metatarsal is more angulated than are the other four, but all are angulated.
7. The talus is medially and anteriorly displaced in its relationship to the calcaneus.
8. There is no equinus or any limitation of dorsiflexion as seen in talipes equinovarus.

Metatarsus varus is not a severe deformity, but the child may walk in an awkward manner with toeing in and tripping over his or her own feet.

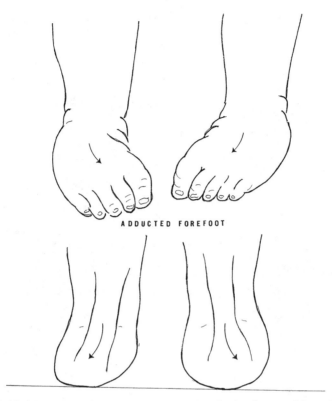

ADDUCTED FOREFOOT

**Figure 4–12.** Metatarsus varus. In metatarsus varus, the foot has an adducted forefoot, a convex lateral foot border, and the heel is in valgus. There is no equinus.

## Treatment

Treatment should be initiated early, although the condition often does correct itself. In a large percentage of children, however, the condition persists, causing a cosmetic and psychologic impairment and functional disability. If treatment is undertaken, it must be vigorously applied and followed over time. Parental manual treatments are usually inadequate because they cannot be done often enough. Therefore, the benefit gained is not held, and the condition may even progress.

A Denis Browne splint has enjoyed use, but it has the danger of everting the feet, thus accentuating the heel valgus without correcting the forefoot (Fig. 4–14).

Reversing the shoes, the left on the right, and vice versa, may hold and even correct the very mild metatarsus varus, but this does not correct the more moderate or severe varus.

A series of correcting plaster casts usually corrects the forefoot and the hindfoot, if properly applied. The technique of plaster casting is the technique of correction (Fig. 4–15). The heel is forced medially (varus), thus moving the

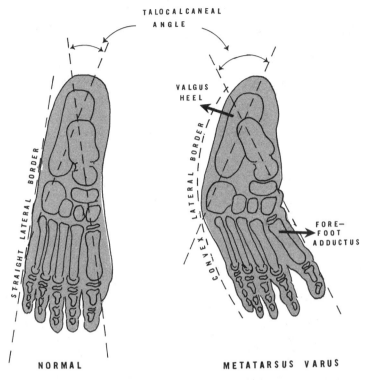

**Figure 4–13.** Metatarsus varus compared to the normal foot. The metatarsus varus foot has an adducted forefoot, a valgus heel, and a convexly curved lateral border with its apex at the base of the fifth metatarsal. The talus is medially and anteriorly displaced in relationship to the calcaneus, thus increasing the talocalcaneal angle.

calcaneus under the talus. This requires pressure on the cuboid while simultaneously moving the calcaneus and forefoot into adduction.

The cast should be applied to the foot in a slight equinus and slight inversion to the long axis of the leg. The toes should remain exposed. The foot correction can be better maintained if the cast extends above the knee, which thus also permits a slight correction of the tibial torsion.

After casting and before the cast is dry, the transverse metatarsal arch is molded into a slight dorsal convexity. Each cast should be left on for 2 weeks before recorrecting and recasting. Ultimately the foot should be slightly "overcorrected" since some correction is usually lost.

This condition must not be confused with the more serious talipes equinovarus ("clubfoot"). In metatarsus varus, the heel is in valgus positions, whereas in talipes equinovarus, the heel is in varus (Fig. 4–16). In a clubfoot, the foot is in equinus and resists dorsiflexion because of a contracted gastrocnemius-

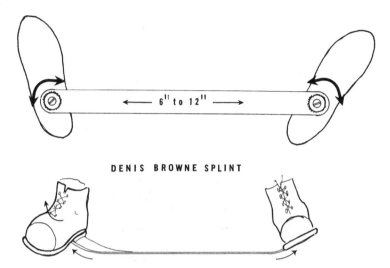

**Figure 4–14.** The Denis Browne splint. A spreader bar, which may be metal, wood, or plastic, is firmly attached to the soles of each shoe. This attachment is adjustable so that the shoe may be turned out to any desired angle. The bar may be bent at its ends to evert or invert the shoe. The width of the spreader bar varies with the age and size of the child, and the angles vary according to the desired correction of the feet and lower leg(s).

soleus muscle and Achilles tendon. This is not present in metatarsus varus, where the heel can usually be easily moved and the foot readily dorsiflexed.

## METATARSUS PRIMUS VARUS

*Metatarsus primus varus* simulates metatarsus varus since the forefoot appears to be adducted, but in this condition only the first metatarsal bone is in varus and the other toes are in proper alignment (Fig. 4–17). The first metatarsal angulates medially on the medial cuneiform or may be aligned properly on a deformed cuneiform. The lateral foot margin shows no convexity, as is noted in metatarsus varus. Radiologic diagnosis confirms this condition.

Treatment is usually unnecessary since this deformity causes no symptoms other than possibly predisposing to a hallux valgus (to be discussed).

## TALIPES EQUINOVARUS
## (CONGENITAL CLUBFOOT)

This is a relatively common condition and is considered one of the "big three" congenital conditions: congenital hip dislocation, myelomeningocele, and clubfoot. Talipes equinovarus was first described in ancient times by Hippocrates.[5] It

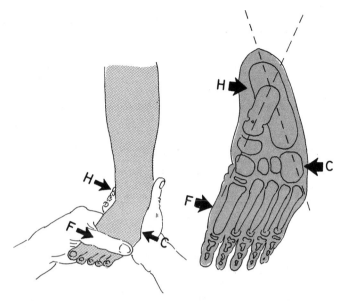

**Figure 4–15.** Technique of manually correcting metatarsus varus before plaster casting. Pressure C is applied against the cuboid bone and the anterior portion of the calcaneus medially, forcing the calcaneus under the talus. This corrects the valgus heel. H is traction on the posterior calcaneus to aid C in moving the calcaneus into a neutral position. F is simultaneous pressure using the other hand to correct the adducted metatarsals. All pressures shown must be applied simultaneously.

has an incidence of 1 per 1000 live births, with 1.2 per 1000 in Caucasians and nearly a 2 to 1 male to female predominance.[6–8] It has a higher incidence in full-blooded Hawaiians,[9] South African Blacks,[10] and Polynesians.[11] It is bilateral in 50% of cases and, when unilateral, is on the side of predominance.[12]

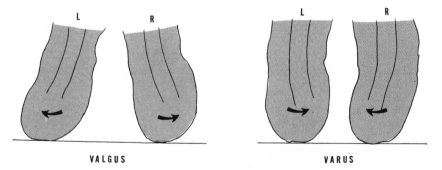

**Figure 4–16.** Valgus-varus heels. As seen from behind in weight bearing, the right foot (R) and left foot (L) have visible heel alignment, which differentiates metatarsus varus from talipes equinovarus (see accompanying text).

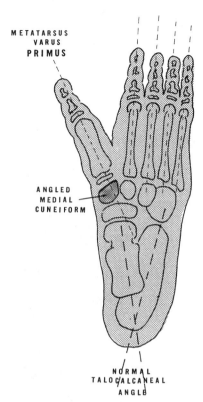

**Figure 4–17.** Metatarsus primus varus. Metatarsus primus varus grossly resembles metatarsus varus, but in primus only the first metatarsal is adducted. The remaining metatarsals are in proper alignment. The first metatarsal may adduct because of a deformed medial cuneiform or may be angled medially on a normal cuneiform. The talocalcaneal angle reveals no deviation of the talar relationship on the calcaneus.

## Diagnosis

The condition is characterized by the following components: (1) inversion (twisting inward) and adduction (inward deviation) of the forefoot (Fig. 4–18); (2) varus of the calcaneus (inversion of the heel); (3) equinus (plantar flexion); (4) contraction of the tissues on the medial side of the foot; (5) underdeveloped everter muscles of the lateral side of the lower leg; (6) underdeveloped and contracted calf muscles; and (7) resistance to passive manual correction.

A plantar-flexed, inverted foot in a newborn that cannot easily be brought into a dorsiflexed and/or everted position suggests talipes equinovarus. This is contrary to the normal child, in whom the foot may be plantar-flexed and inverted but is flexible and can be easily corrected. It also differs from the metatarsus varus foot, in which the forefoot is in varus but the heel is in valgus and is mobile.

In talipes equinovarus (clubfoot), the toes are also flexed and resist passive extension. There is also an associated internal tibial torsion. The child stands bearing weight on the base of the fifth metatarsal bone.

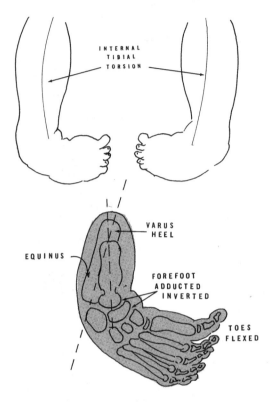

**Figure 4–18.** Talipes equinovarus: "Clubfoot." Talipes equinovarus or "clubfoot" has an inflexible adducted forefoot and a varus heel. The toes are usually flexed, and the medial soft tissues are contracted. The Achilles tendon is shortened, and there is usually an internal tibial torsion. All these deformities resist passive stretching and elongation.

## Etiology

There are many theories regarding the etiology of talipes equinovarus, but none is without controversy. Originally, Hippocrates considered intrauterine mechanical pressures from intrauterine malposition.[13] The condition has been considered as being transmitted by means of mandelian patterns and even X-linked with chromosomal abnormalities, but this will remain for future geneticists to postulate.

## Pathoanatomic Factors

With the presence of talipes equinovarus, the pathoanatomic aspects must be understood and addressed in its management.

The chief abnormality is a deformity of the talus, which is smaller than normal and has a plantar and medial deviation of the head and neck. The calcaneus and navicular are displaced around the deformed talus in a plantar and medial direction. The talus adapts within the ankle mortise since the navicular abuts the medial malleolus.

Soft-tissue contractures serve to prevent spontaneous rearrangement[14,15] and hold the bony malposition, while the muscular deficiencies fail to exert corrective forces.[16] It is apparent from all pathoanatomic studies that this condition is more complex than merely a primary bony[17] deformity, and all ligaments, capsular and muscular, have to be addressed in its management.

## Treatment and Management

The foot initially must be manipulated with gentle stretching followed by taping and/or castings. Improper and excessive stretching can result in a foot that is less functional.[18,19] Conservative treatment will correct about one-third to one-half of congenital clubfeet, but only the milder cases.[13,20,21] Treatment should be initiated, however, and held by casting, awaiting more definitive surgery. Surgical intervention as early as the first week has been disappointing.[22] Beginning surgical intervention at 3 to 6 months is considered the ideal age,[23] in that the maximum remodeling potential is best achieved while the still-cartilaginous tarsal bone remains. Before that age, the infant's structures are too small, causing technical difficulties. After age 12 months, there is a significant loss of remodeling potential.

Surgical techniques are not the basis of this text. Suffice it to say that the surgical procedures are essentially soft-tissue release or lengthening or both in order to correct the adduction of the forefoot, release the Achilles tendon (correct the equinus), and release the capsular tissues that have immobilized the various joints so discovered. Careful postoperative management helps achieve a pain-free, functional, and cosmetically acceptable foot (feet).

## TARSAL COALITION

Rigid flatfoot is frequently caused by an anomalous fusion of two or more tarsal bones.[24,25] This coalition prevents movement between the two involved tarsal bones, causing a static foot deformity. The fusion may be osseous, cartilaginous, or fibrous. The most common coalitions exist between the talus and the calcaneus or between the calcaneus and the navicular (Fig. 4–19).

## Diagnosis

Tarsal coalitions may be asymptomatic. They probably exist from birth and rarely give symptoms until late adolescence or early adulthood when

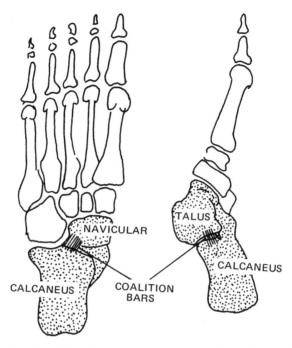

**Figure 4–19.** Tarsal coalition. Tarsal coalition is an anomalous fusion of two or more tarsal bones by a bony, cartilaginous, or fibrous bar. The most common types are tarso-calcaneal and/or calcaneonavicular. Their presence may form a rigid flatfoot or a peroneal "spastic" flatfoot. When the bar is bone, it can be visualized on x-ray; otherwise, its presence is diagnosed clinically.

superimposed trauma such as prolonged standing, marching, or jumping induces symptoms. The pain undoubtedly results from stress sustained by the remaining unfused joints that are excessively moved as a result of the fused ones.

X-rays are diagnostic if the fusion is osseous but are not in cartilage or fibrous fusion. Diagnosis here must be clinical suspicion by manual testing of all joints of the foot.

## Treatment

Treatment is supportive, depending on the severity. If the condition is very acute and severe, immobilization in a cast may afford relief and yet permit weight bearing and ambulation. If persistent and disabling, surgical removal of the bar may be considered with or without fusion of the symptomatic joints.

# CONGENITAL VERTICAL TALUS

This is an uncommon condition but should be suspected when the foot of the newborn is fixed in equinus *and* abduction. When the foot is passively dorsiflexed, the head of the talus forms a prominence at the expected longitudinal arch concavity, forming a "rocker-bottom" foot.[26] This may resemble a clubfoot. X-rays reveal the vertical talus.

## Treatment

Treating this condition by manipulation and then casting is warranted but usually disappointing in that the foot appears improved but is not necessarily painlessly functional. Surgical correction offers the most benefit.

## REFERENCES

1. Gartland, JJ: Fundamentals of Orthopaedics. WB Saunders, Philadelphia, 1965.
2. MacConail, MA: The postural mechanism of the human foot. Proc Roy Irish Acad 1B:265, May 1945.
3. Goldner, JL: Congenital talipes equinovarus—Fifteen years of surgical treatment. Curr Prac Orthop Surg 4:16–123, 1969.
4. Drvaric, DM, Kuivila, TE, and Roberts, JM: Congenital clubfoot: Etiology, pathoanatomy, pathogenesis and the changing spectrum of early management. Ortho Clin North Am 20(4): 641–647, 1989.
5. Hippocrates: Loeb Classical Library, Vol. 3. Withington, ET (transl). William Heinemann, Ltd, London, and GP Putnam, New York, 1927.
6. Wynne-Davies, R: Family studies and cause of congenital club foot. J Bone Joint Surg 46B:445, 1964.
7. Wynne-Davies, R: Heritable disorders in orthopaedic practice. Oxford, Blackwell Scientific Publications, 1973, p 206.
8. Wynne-Davies, R: The genetics of some common congenital malformations. In Emery, A (ed): Modern Trends in Human Genetics. Butterworths, London, 1970, chap 11.
9. Stewart, SF: Club foot: Its incidence, cause and treatment. Anatomical physiologic study. J Bone Joint Surg 33A:577, 1951.
10. Pompe van Meerdervoort, HP: Congenital musculoskeletal disorders in the South African negro. J Bone Joint Surg 59B:257, 1977.
11. Pillay, VK, Khong, BT, and Wolfers, D: The inheritance of club foot in Singapore. Proc Third Malaysian Congress of Medicine 3:102, 1967.
12. Palmer, RM, Conneally, PM, and Yu, PL: Studies of the inheritance of ideopathic talipes equinovarus. Orthop Clin North Am 5:99, 1974.
13. Tachdjian, MO (ed): Congenital deformities: Congenital talipes equinovarus. In The Child's Foot. WB Saunders, Philadelphia, 1985, pp 139–170.
14. Adams, RD, Denny-Brown, D, and Pearson, CM: Diseases of Muscle: A Study in Pathology, ed 2. Harper and Brothers, New York, 1962, p 304.
15. Smith, RD: Dysplasia and the effects of soft tissue release in congenital talipes equinovarus. Clin Orthop 174:303–309, 1983.

16. Attenborough, CG: Early posterior soft tissue release in severe congenital talipes equinovarus. Clin Orthop 84:71, 1972.
17. Ponset, IV, and Campus J: Observations on pathogenesis and treatment of congenital clubfoot. Clin Orthop 84:50, 1972.
18. Simons, GW: Complete subtalar release in club feet: Part I. A preliminary report. J Bone Joint Surg 67A:1044, 1985.
19. Simons, GW: Complete subtalar release in club feet. Part II. Comparison with less extensive procedures. J Bone Joint Surg 67A:1056, 1985.
20. Goldner, JL: Congenital talipes equinovarus: Fifteen years of surgical treatment. Cur Prac Orthop Surg 4:61–123, 1969.
21. Kaski, T, and Wosko, I: Experience in the conservative treatment of congenital clubfoot in newborns and infants. J Pediatr Orthop 9:134, 1989.
22. Ryoppy, S, and Sairane, H: Neonatal operative treatment of club foot: A preliminary report. J Bone Joint Surg 65B:320, 1983.
23. Thompson, GH, Richardson, AB, and Westin, GW: Surgical management of resisted congenital talipes equinovarus deformities. J Bone Joint Surg 64A:652–665, 1982.
24. Vaughn, WH, and Segal, G: Tarsal coalition with special reference to roentgenographic interpretation. Radiology 60:855, 1953.
25. Webster, FS, and Roberts, WM: Tarsal anomalies and peroneal spastic flatfoot. JAMA 146:1099, 1951.
26. Hark, FW: Rocker-foot due to congenital subluxation of the talus. J Bone Joint Surg 32A:344, 1950.

# CHAPTER 5

# Painful Disorders of the Adult Foot

The *normal foot* must conform to the following criteria: (1) be pain-free, (2) have normal muscle balance, (3) have an absence of contracture, (4) have three-point weight bearing during stance and gait, (5) have a central heel, and (6) have straight and mobile toes.

The majority of painful conditions in the adult foot originate in soft tissues[1]: the muscles, ligaments, tendons, joint capsules, nerves, and blood vessels. Articular and skeletal causes may be present from congenital abnormalities, infections, neoplasms, and/or trauma. Regardless of the etiology, the early symptoms and impairment come from soft-tissue changes.

As in all neuromusculoskeletal dysfunctions, the same adage applies: pain and dysfunction can occur from (1) abnormal stress on a normal structure, (2) normal stress on an abnormal structure, and (3) normal stress on a normal structure that is not, at that moment, prepared for the imposed stress. More recently, a fourth can be added: (4) "repetitive" stresses that are otherwise normal on normal tissues can lead to pain and dysfunction.

The static foot is supported by ligamentous and congruous tissue. There is no muscular activity in the foot or leg during stance, even when large weights are superimposed on the body. Minor deviation from the center of gravity does cause an instantaneous burst of muscular activities in a *righting reflex* that disappears on return to the center of gravity position.

The foot is essentially balanced by congruity of the composing bones and their joints, their capsules, and the ligaments. Besides initiating a right reflex, muscular activity prevents excessive stress on the supporting ligaments and joint tissues. Faulty function imposed on the static foot during locomotion may result in pain and dysfunction.

Muscular incompetence from disease, disuse, abuse, or imbalance can place excessive stress on ligaments and articular surfaces, resulting in inflammation, tissue damage, and ultimate degeneration.

The history gained from the patient is unique in foot pain as compared to other neuromusculoskeletal conditions in that the history alludes to the cause of the subsequent pain and impairment, and the patient can precisely point to "the" anatomic site of the painful tissue. Occasionally, "foot pain" is a referred manifestation of pathology elsewhere referred to the foot. Properly and carefully undertaken, the history and examination reveal this condition.

Many foot conditions such as pronation may be present but may not necessarily be painful or disabling and may not be the basis for the presenting complaints of the patient.

## FOOT STRAIN

The foot that has been *strained* may be classified as acute, subacute, or chronic. Strain is essentially mechanical force imposed on "soft" tissue that causes deformation termed sprain. Strain is injury caused by too strong an effort or from excessive use. Sprain[2] is injury to a joint that causes pain and disability with deformation of collagen tissue.[3]

### Acute Foot Strain

Acute foot strain is encountered after prolonged standing, walking, running, or jumping that has not been previously undertaken. The pain is noted in ligaments, tendons, muscles, joints, or even the periosteum of the offended bones. Ambulation in a strange and uneven terrain may be the offender, and faulty footwear may also be responsible. This is an example of "normal" stress on a normal foot where normal stress is excessive and abnormal in intensity or frequency.

Examination reveals evidence of "inflammation" by erythema, edema, acute callous, or localized tissue tenderness. Radiologic studies are usually unnecessary unless a stress fracture is suspected. Local remedies such as rest, elevation, modalities of ice and/or heat, and anti-inflammatory medication usually suffice.

### Chronic Foot Strain

If excessive stress is repeated or if normal stress that is required during daily activities is imposed on a structurally damaged foot, chronic pain results. Pain will remain or recur on resumption of the activity. Pain occurs from tissues nociceptively endowed being stressed beyond their resilience. If the stress is excessive or repetitive, the "normal" deformation of the stressed tissue that should recover does not occur, and there results persistent deformation (Figs. 5–1 and 5–2).

Pain that results becomes programmed within the central nervous system, enhancing the severity and persistence of the pain. It may lead to chronic pain even when peripheral nociceptors are no longer being stimulated (Fig. 5–3).[4]

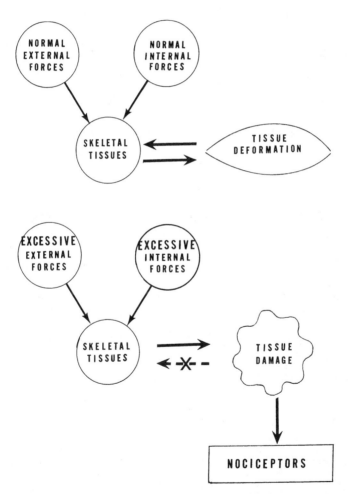

**Figure 5–1.** Normal and excessive forces on the musculoskeletal system. *Upper diagram:* Normal external and internal forces on the musculoskeletal tissues causing reversible deformation. Resultant pain and dysfunction are not expected. *Lower diagram:* Excessive forces on the skeletal tissues causing irreversible damage with release of nociceptor elements. Pain and dysfunction result.

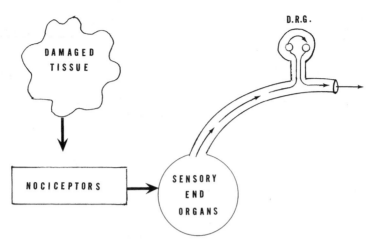

**Figure 5–2.** Sequence of tissue damage creating nociceptors. The injured tissues liberate chemical nociceptors that inflame (irritate) the sensory end organs, releasing impulses to the dorsal root ganglia (DRG) via C unmyelinated and A alpha fibers, initiating ultimate pain perception.

The tissue breakdown that occurs from repeated stress or from stress on abnormal tissues follows a sequence. Ligaments, tendons, and capsular tissue exposed to chronic stress undergo elongation beyond their mutability. *Stress* refers to the amount of tension or load per unit, and strain refers to the proportional elongation that results.[3]

Because ligaments are attached to bone, tension within them can build up when they are stretched by a change in the geometry of the joints in which they are involved. Because ligaments are composed of parallel fibers, they can be stretched only by 6 to 8% of their rest length.

This stress-strain curve involves five distinct regions in the tendon or ligament:

*Toe region*: Little increase in stress with elongation; 1.2 to 1.5% strain effect; within physiologic limits.

*Linear region*: Stress rapidly increases with increased elongation; microfailure begins.

*Progressive failure region*: In spite of appearing normal to the naked eye, disruption of the tissue occurs.

*Major failure region*: Tendon remains intact but narrows at points of shear, and ruptures are visible.

*Complete rupture region*: Gross tendon breaks.

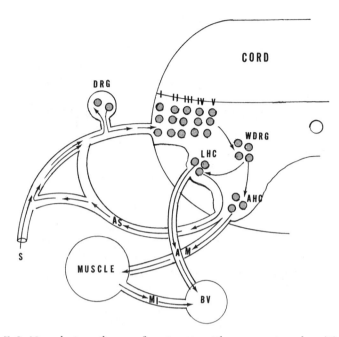

**Figure 5–3.** Neurologic pathways of nociception. The sensory impulses (S) enter via afferent fibers to the dorsal root ganglion (DRG) then to the Rexed layers I, II, III, IV, V, and so on. Layers I and II are the substantia gelatinosa. Intraneural fibers then transmit impulses to the lateral spinothalamic tracts (not shown) to the hypothalamus, the thalamus, and ultimately the cortex. Nociceptive impulses transmit to the wide-dynamic-range ganglia (WDRG) to the lateral horn cells (LHC), which initiate autonomic impulses, and to the anterior horn cells (AHC), which initiate muscular response. The efferent fibers from LHC innervate the blood vessels (BV) in the area of nociception. Afferent autonomic fibers transmit sensation (AS) to the DRG. The skeletal muscles innervated by efferents (AM) from AHC cause ischemia of the muscles from persistent excessive contraction, causing autonomic impulses (MI) from the involved blood vessels. See the accompanying text for details of these pathways.

These regions of injury apply to tendons and/or ligaments and even to collagen within capsules and are visible and clinically apparent only in later stages (regions).

As the ligaments elongate and degenerate, they lose their protective supportive function and permit excessive motion of the joint. Their proprioceptive function is also impaired.[5,6] Excessive "play" and misalignment of the joint inflame the joint capsule and its articular surfaces. This inflammation becomes a site and source of pain. Gradually, degenerative changes in the cartilage occur (Figs. 5–4 through 5–7).

If irritation to the joint continues, structural damage to the articular surfaces result with the onset of *degenerative* arthritic changes. These changes, termed *arthrosis*, are attempts of repair by nature (Fig. 5–8). Early recognition

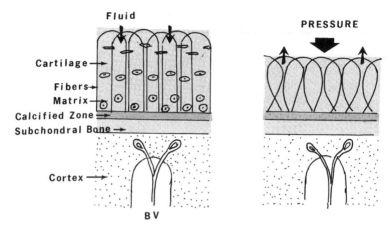

**Figure 5–4.** Nutrition of cartilage. The blood supply to cartilage in bone cortex comes only to the subchondral layer. As pressure is applied to cartilage and then released, the release "imbibes" nutrition from the blood that penetrates the subchondral bone

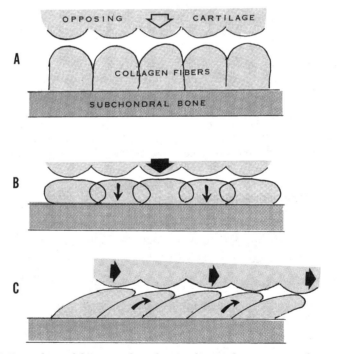

**Figure 5–5.** Mechanical function of cartilage. *A* depicts the structures of opposing cartilages. The coiled collagen acts as "springs" that compress (*B*) when under pressure. This forces fluid within the cartilage to enter the subchondral bone. Upon release (not shown) the cartilage "imbibes" joint fluid. (*C*) On lateral shear the cartilage deforms but retains its basic structure.

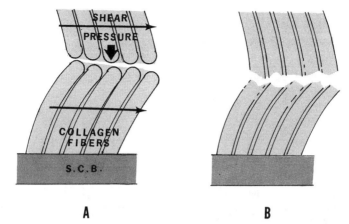

**A**                                    **B**

**Figure 5–6.** Progressive cartilage changes. The left figure (*A*) indicates the reversible changes that occur to the collagen fibers during compression and shear in which the coiled fibers retain their configuration. In *B*, after excessive or traumatic injury, the coiled collagen fibers are broken and lose their reversibility. The cartilage is now denied its inhibitory facilities and begins degenerative changes.

and intervention may impede arthritic progress before irreversible changes occur.

The initial symptoms of chronic pain from predisposing activity are usually muscular fatigue described as "aching" in the muscles of the foot and/or lower leg. Deep tenderness is elicited in the inflamed tissues. Continued, aggravating activity changes the symptoms from muscular fatigue and ache to tendinous-ligamentous pain. Points of localized tenderness may be elicited by palpation over the periosteal tissues of the offended bones where tendons insert (Fig. 5–9).

## Mechanisms of Symptomatic Foot Strain

The foot must be considered as a complex structure with each component part dependent on the other adjacent structures. The talus bears the total body

**Figure 5–7.** Basis of synovitis. When there is joint injury or inflammation, the synovium enlarges and forms a "pannus" (*A*), which coats the cartilage. There is also migration of the inflamed synovium that invades the space between the cartilage and its subchondral bone-impairing nutrition.

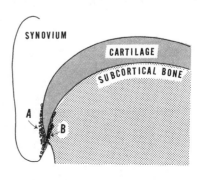

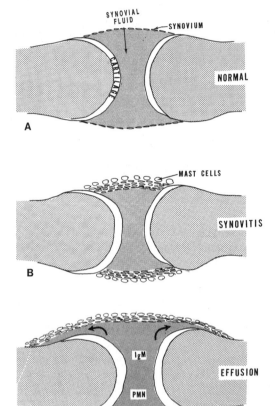

**Figure 5–8.** Stages of joint degenerative disease. *A* depicts a normal joint. With inflammation from injury or disease, the synovium enlarges and is filled with mast cells (*B*), which create IgM (*C*) and lysozymes, which "digest" the cartilage (*D*). Ultimately, the cartilage becomes denuded with subcortical atrophy (*E*), and fibrous tissue invades the joint, uniting the opposing denuded bones. (*continued on next page*)

weight through its articulation within the mortise formed by the tibia and fibula. The talus in turn is borne by the calcaneus in an oblique manner (Fig. 5–10) and stabilized by a ligamentous complex (Fig. 5–11). The oblique seating of the talus on the calcaneus gives the talus a tendency to glide forward and medially upon the calcaneus (Fig. 5–12). This forces the calcaneus into eversion and depresses the anterior portion. The resultant pronation depresses the longitudinal arch, stretching the plantar ligament and the fascia.

The valgus position of the heel places a torque stress on the forefoot, which responds by everting. The foot now bears the weight on the inner border, which forces the foot to evert more into pronation, placing strain on the medial ankle ligaments and on the posterior tibialis tendon. Because of the valgus position of the heel, the gastrocnemius-soleus tendon deviates laterally and gradually shortens, placing more strain on the anterior segments of the foot.

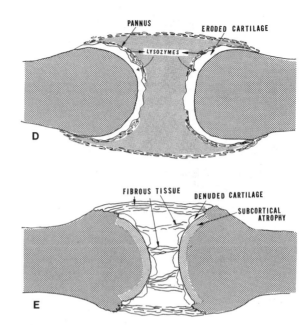

Figure 5–8   (*continued*)

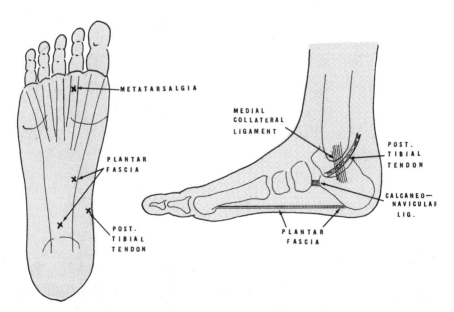

**Figure 5–9.** Tender areas in foot strain. All the soft tissues that become tender from foot strain are pointed to by the patient and palpable by the examiner.

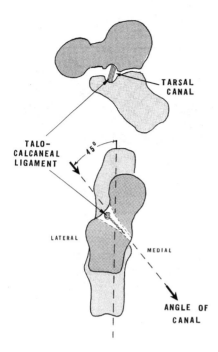

TARSAL CANAL

TALO-CALCANEAL LIGAMENT

LATERAL

MEDIAL

45°

ANGLE OF CANAL

**Figure 5–10.** Talocalcaneal joint. The talus and calcaneus are joined by three facets: anterior, middle, and posterior. The tarsal tunnel in its oblique course (sulcus) contains the talocalcaneal ligaments.

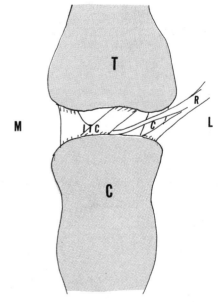

**Figure 5–11.** Ligamentous complex of the talocalcaneal joint. The talus (T) and calcaneus (C) form the talocalcaneal joint. It is connected by a capsule (not shown) and the interosseous talocalcaneal ligament (ITC), cervical (c) ligament, and retinaculum (R).

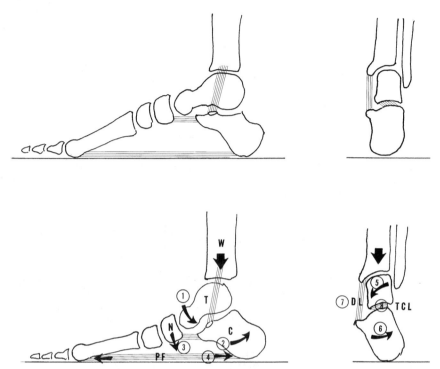

**Figure 5–12.** Mechanism of foot strain. *Upper figures* depict the normal foot seen laterally (*left*) and posteriorly (*right*). There is a good longitudinal arch and a central heel. Lower figures show weight bearing (W) upon malaligned foot structures, which causes the talus (T) to glide forward (1) and medially (5) and the calcaneus (C) to rotate posteriorly (2), placing strain on the calcaneonavicular ligament. The navicular (N) is depressed (3). The flattening of the longitudinal arch places stress upon the plantar fascia (PF) (4). The resultant pronation causes the heel to evert (6) placing strain on the medial deltoid ligament (DL) (7) and the talocalcaneal ligament (TCL) (8).

## Diagnosis

The sequence of foot strain may be manifested on the normal foot but is more apt to occur in a deconditioned foot and especially in the already pronated foot. Normally, there is protective muscular action on the foot, but as stress is imparted, the muscles fail and the stress is inflicted on the ligaments and ultimately the joint capsules. As the ligaments undergo changes, initially reversible, these changes become irreversible and joint deformation occurs.

As capsular changes occur, they too, being essentially collagen in structure, go from reversible to irreversible. The joints that normally are essentially stable by virtue of being congruous now become more incongruous and thus unstable. Structural changes occur where there is cartilage and where there is significant structural incongruity.

## Stages

During the early phase of foot stress and strain, the muscles attempt to allay the strain on the ligaments and the joint capsules. The proprioceptive receptors within these soft tissues[5,6] assure appropriate muscular contraction. When there is inappropriate and prolonged muscular contraction, fatigue and thus muscular pain result.

The posterior tibialis muscle is the prime *invertor* that opposes pronation, which is functionally *eversion*. The posterior tibialis tendon may become inflamed and tender with other signs of inflammation. When the pronation remains uncorrected, pain is elicited during prolonged stance and prolonged walking.

On examination, tenderness can be palpated in the region under and behind the medial malleolous (see Fig. 5–9). The long flexor of the big toe may also be strained and painfully inflamed as it functions in a manner similar to the posterior tibialis as well as pressing the toe to the ground during gait.

As the strain persists and the forefoot goes into more pronation, the lateral evertors, the peronei, and the toe extensors shorten to take up the slack. This "shortening" indicates sustained muscular contraction with local tenderness.

## Examination of the Strained Foot

As a history of pain related to the foot and ankle is elicited, the examination must now determine which tissue is responsible for the pain and impairment. As has been stated, the foot is amenable to direct examination after the patient has pointed to where the foot hurts and indicated when it hurts.

The interosseous talocalcaneal, which binds the talus to the calcaneus, is normally taut when the foot is supinated, but in pronation becomes slack (Fig. 5–13). This permits separation of the two bones, causing deformation of the tarsal tunnel with resultant inflammation of the interosseous ligament. This tenderness is elicited digitally at the lateral orifice of the sinus canal just anterior to the lateral malleolus with the foot passively inverted (Fig. 5–14). This is a late sequela in foot strain of the pronated foot.

In the pronated foot, there is also usually a flattening of the longitudinal arch. In foot strain, the plantar fascia becomes stretched, and tenderness and pain are noted in the bottom of the foot, usually at the anterior portion of the calcaneus (Fig. 5–15). As the plantar fascia attaches to the periosteum of the calcaneus, it can easily be palpated (Fig. 5–16).

The ligaments, specifically those in the heel region, must also be tested as being the tissue site of pain. In a severe stress-strain of the hind foot and in chronic pain after the injury, the talocalcaneal joint must be tested to determine the adequacy of the talocalcaneal ligament (see Fig. 5–11). This is done by placing the foot in extreme dorsiflexion, which places the anterior, and wider, por-

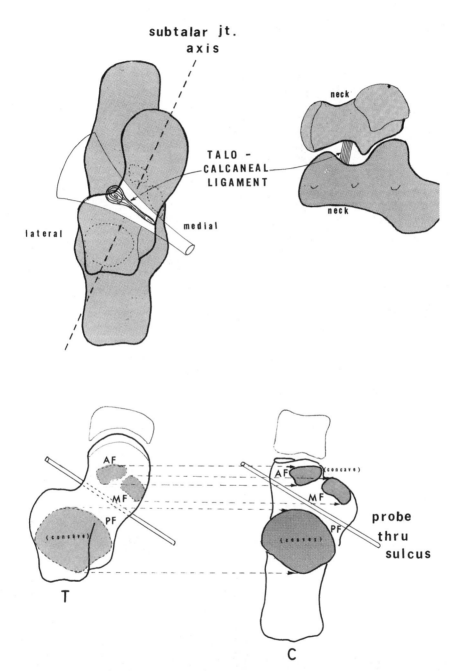

**Figure 5–13.** Talocalcaneal ligament. The talus and calcaneus are joined by three facets: AF, anterior; MF, middle; and PF, posterior. The sinus tarsi (tarsal canal) in its oblique course contains the talocalcaneal ligament, which binds the two bones.

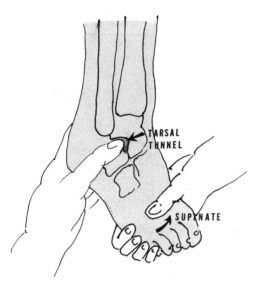

**Figure 5–14.** Palpation of the tarsal tunnel. Palpation below and behind the lateral malleolus with the forefoot supinated exposes the opening to the tarsal tunnel in which is the talocalcaneal ligament.

tion of the talus within the mortise, which immobilizes this joint. The hind foot (calcaneus) is then mobilized by the examiner, who tests the talocalcaneal ligament (Fig. 5–17).

In a pronated foot, the posterior tibial tendon is placed under stretch and thus stress. The patient complains of pain and tenderness in the medial aspect

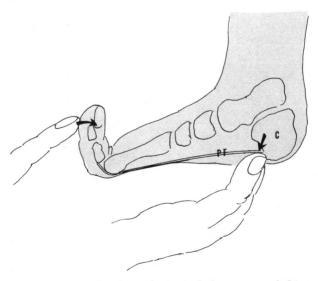

**Figure 5–15.** Palpation of tender plantar fascia. With the toes extended (curved arrow), the plantar fascia is tender where it attaches (straight arrow) to the anterior aspect of the calcaneus (C).

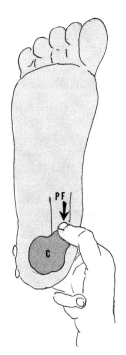

**Figure 5–16.** Palpation of the medial tubercle of the calcaneus. The medial tubercle of the calcaneus (C) is the site of attachment of the plantar fascia (PF) and, medially, the abductor hallucis and origin of the flexor digitorum brevis (not shown). The medial tubercle is the weight-bearing point on the calcaneus during gait.

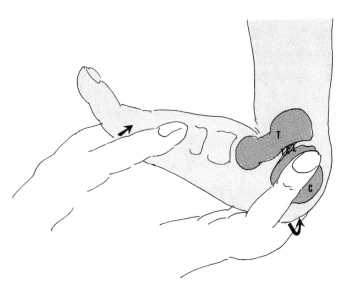

**Figure 5–17.** Testing talocalcaneal stability. By dorsiflexing the foot (straight arrow, left hand), the talus (T) becomes "locked" within the ankle mortise as the anterior portion of the body of the talus becomes wedged between the medial and lateral malleoli. Mobilization of the calcaneus (C) (curved arrow) tests the talocalcaneal ligament (TCL) and joint stability.

of the foot, which is aggravated when the foot is placed in eversion or when the foot is actively placed in plantar flexion and inversion, which is the primary function of the posterior tibial muscle-tendon complex. Examination of this patient requires eliciting tenderness in the posterior tibial tendon and the spring ligament (Fig. 5–18).

At the heel, the Achilles tendon is also subject to stress-strain. This is increasingly prevalent in today's society of weekend athletes. The injury is usually forceful because this tendon is resilient. This history alludes to the injury, which may be "internal" stress such as forceful, repeated jumping and excessive stress of the elongated tendon, or it can result from an extrernal blow to the tendon.

With the foot plantar flexed or dorsiflexed, the Achilles tendon can be examined by manually palpating it (Fig. 5–19). The patient usually also has pain and weakness on rising up on his or her toes.

The gastrocnemius muscle must also be examined. This can easily be done with the patient kneeling on a flat surface and the foot extending over the edge. The calf muscle (gastrocnemius muscle) is amenable to palpation (Fig. 5–20). This can be performed with the foot dorsiflexed or actively plantar flexed. If the Achilles tendon is totally torn, squeezing the gastrocnemius muscle does not plantar flex the foot, as normally occurs.

If there is an acute bursitis of the bursae between the Achilles tendon and the tibia or superficial to the tendon, this is usually visible as inflamed swelling that is tender to palpation (Fig. 5–21).

When the tissue site has been pinpointed as the site of trauma and nociception, a means of management must then be determined.

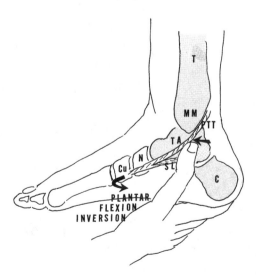

**Figure 5–18.** Palpation of the posterior tibial tendon and spring ligament. The posterior tibialis tendon (PTT) and spring ligament (SL) can be palpated behind and beneath the medial malleolus (MM) of the tibia (T). The tendon becomes activated when the foot is actively plantar flexed and inverted. The tendon attaches to the navicular (N), which articulates with the cuneiform (Cu) and the talus (TA). The calcaneus (C) is also shown.

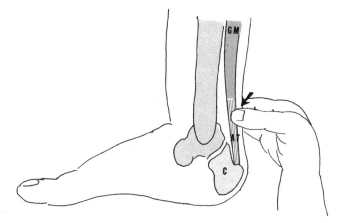

**Figure 5–19.** Palpation of the Achilles tendon. The Achilles tendon (AT) can be palpated between the thumb and the index finger just superior to the calcaneus (C). Normally, if the pressure is excessive, it is tender; but it is also sensitive to moderate pressure, as compared to the other side, in the presence of tendinitis or partial tearing of the collagen fibers.

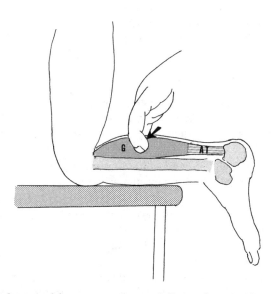

**Figure 5–20.** Palpation of the gastrocnemius-Achilles tendon complex. With the patient kneeling, as shown, the gastrocnemius muscle can be palated for tenderness during plantar flexion of the foot, which normally occurs when the Achilles tendon is intact. If there is a gastrocnemius strain or even muscle fiber tears, this will elicit tenderness. If there is a complete tear of the Achilles tendon, the foot will not plantar flex on gastrocnemius squeezing.

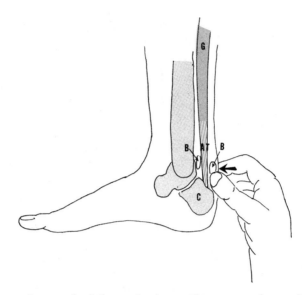

**Figure 5–21.** Palpation of Achilles tendon bursa. There are two bursae (B) in the heel region. One exists between the Achilles tendon and the tibia, and the other between the Achilles tendon and the underlying skin. Either can become inflamed when there is pressure, direct trauma, or friction, usually from a shoe counter. Bursae usually cannot be palpated, but when inflamed and swollen, they appear on visual examination and can be palpated. Once the Achilles tendon is palpated (see Fig. 5–19), the precise bursa can be determined.

If pain occurring at the heel is noted, this can be evaluated as being plantar fasciitis, bursitis, tendinitis, possible fracture, or periostitis. The tissue site can be ascertained by careful digital pressure that reproduces the pain.

The chronically strained foot, usually the pronated, everted forefoot, places stress on any or all the joints of the foot anterior to the talus. The patient points to the specific joint and the examiner determines the site and the presence of the pathology (Fig. 5–22). Radiologic studies are diagnostic only after there has been degeneration of the articular surfaces of that particular joint. Each joint can be palpated.

In a patient with a hallux valgus, there also may be articular pain at the first cuneiform-metatarsal joint. The cuboid bone can be palpated, as can the configuration of the cuneiform-metatarsal joint (Fig. 5–23). Mobility and pain production from the cuneiform-metatarsal joint can be tested by mobilization of that joint (Fig. 5–24).

As examination of the foot proceeds anteriorly into the metatarsal heads and toe areas, precise examination of the individual bones and their joints is also possible. Examination of the big toe could comprise an entire chapter, but examination techniques belong in this chapter.

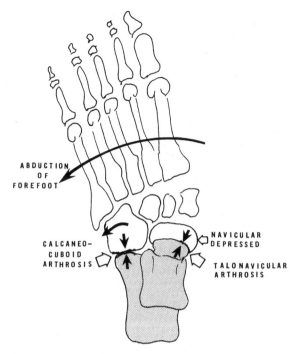

**Figure 5–22.** The chronically strained foot. The abducted forefoot in a chronically strained foot ultimately causes articular changes because of pressure of the abducted cuboid on the calcaneus. The talus drops and causes pressure on the superior portion of the navicular. The articular pressures ultimately cause degeneration, termed *arthrosis*.

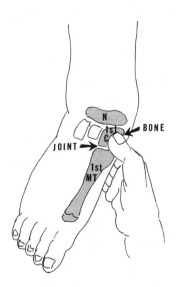

**Figure 5–23.** Palpation of first cuneiform metatarsal joint. Testing of the first cuneiform–first metatarsal joint is shown. The right hand holds the cuneiform (1st C) and the left hand mobilizes the first metatarsal (1st MT).

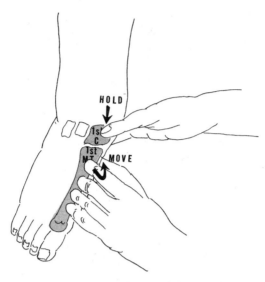

**Figure 5–24.** Palpation of the first cuneiform and the cuneiform-metatarsal joint. The first cuneiform bone and the cuneiform-metatarsal joint can be palpated as shown.

Palpation of the sesamoid bones (Fig. 5–25) is diagnostic when there is weight-bearing pain in that region, with or without hallux valgus, although hallux valgus is usually also present.

In hallux valgus, the first metatarsal proximal phalangeal joint is affected. This joint can be individually examined (Fig. 5–26), both in normally aligned

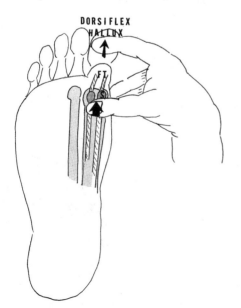

**Figure 5–25.** Palpation of the sesamoid bones. The thumb palpates (large arrow) the sesamoid bones, which are located within the flexor tendons (FT). The tendons are made taut by dorsiflexing the hallux with the index finger (small arrow).

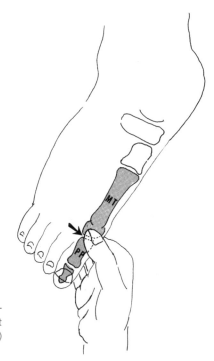

**Figure 5–26.** Palpation of the first metatarsophalangeal joint. Palpation of the first metatarsal (MT)–proximal phalangeal (PP) joint is shown.

first ray or in hallux valgus. Manual mobilization of the first toe indicates the adequacy of the cartilage of that joint (Fig. 5–27). In hallux valgus or degenerative arthritis, there is crepitation, pain, and altered range of motion (either restrictive or excessive mobility). In hallux valgus, besides the varus of the first metatarsal and valgus of the hallux, exostosis is frequently found, as is the presence of an enlarged overlying bursa (Fig. 5–28).

## METATARSALGIA

Metatarsalgia is a well-recognized yet poorly defined pathologic entity.[7] It is essentially a syndrome of pain in the region of the metatarsal heads. It can be acute, recurrent, or chronic and has a host of etiologies that demand a careful, comprehensive evaluation. Causes include vascular, avascular, local mechanical, or neurogenic. Appropriate history and a meaningful examination are again paramount to reaching a specific diagnosis.

### Pain under the Lesser Metatarsals

Pain under the lesser (second, third, and fourth) metatarsals is related to impaired biomechanics of weight bearing. This may be a sequela of faulty gait,

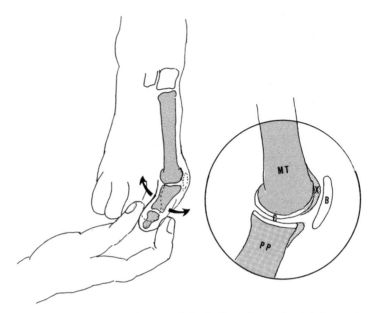

**Figure 5–27.** Mobilization evaluation of the hallux valgus. The *left figure* shows the technique of examination of the first metatarsal (MT) and proximal phalangeal (PP) joint. In this case, it is with hallux valgus, but the examination pertains to examination of a normally aligned joint to determine adequacy of the cartilage (C). In hallux valgus (*right figure*), there is evidence of exostosis (X) and an overlying bursa (B).

iatrogenic from surgical alteration of the foot, congenital, familial, or as a result of deconditioning.

In the pronated foot, the most common *mechanical* basis for metatarsalgia is when the hind foot goes into valgus, the calcaneus deviates on the talus, the forefoot abducts, and the metatarsals widen into a *splayfoot* (Fig. 5–29). This indicates a loss of the normal metatarsal arch, which causes all of the metatarsal heads to bear equal weight (Fig. 5–30). Where normally there is adequate padding over the first and the fifth metatarsal heads and little padding over the other three (Fig. 5–31), now there is equal weight bearing, so that the second, third, and fourth metatarsal heads are exposed to unacceptable pressure.

Pain evidenced over the metatarsal heads is termed *metatarsalgia* (Fig. 5–32). Patients often claim the pain is "like walking with a pebble in the shoe." Ultimately, calluses form over the heads, which aggravates the pressure site.

As the foot further pronates, which it will do since people usually gain some weight with age and their intrinsic muscles lose their tone, the toe extensors function more to dorsiflex the toes, exposing the metatarsal heads to greater pressure (Fig. 5–33).

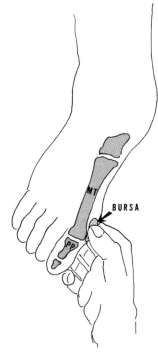

**Figure 5–28.** Examination of bursitis of hallux valgus. An enlarged bursa is frequently palpated in hallux valgus as shown. The first metatarsal (MT) and proximal phalangeal (PP) bones form the metatarsophalangeal joint.

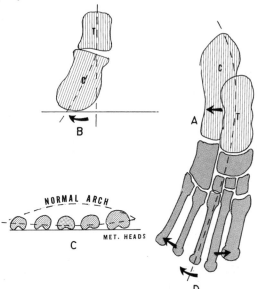

**Figure 5–29.** Aspects of the pronated *splay foot*. *A* shows the valgus position of the calcaneus (C) on the talus (T). This is also displayed in *B. D* shows abduction of the forefoot with separation of the metatarsals (*splay*) causing the metatarsal heads (C) to all bear equal weight.

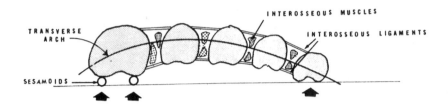

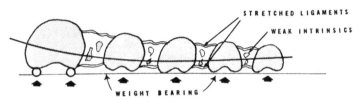

**Figure 5–30.** Splayfoot. A constitutional weakness of the intermetatarsal ligaments combined with weakness of the intrinsic muscles of the foot causes the foot to spread excessively on weight bearing. Symptoms consist of pressure pain on the middle (second, third, and fourth) metatarsal heads with development of bunions and calluses.

## Bunions

Metatarsalgia of the big toe may be related to bunions, arthritis, and sesamoid problems. Pain from bunions usually is related to improper shoe wear and may be associated with hallux valgus, which could constitute an entire chapter.

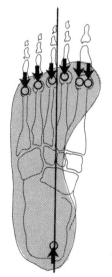

**Figure 5–31.** Weight-bearing points of the foot. There are six weight-bearing points of the metatarsal heads. Because of the two sesamoid bones, the first metatarsal carries two-sixths of the weight. The normal metatarsal arch also assures this balance. A pronated splayfoot disturbs this balance, causing equal weight bearing on all metatarsal heads.

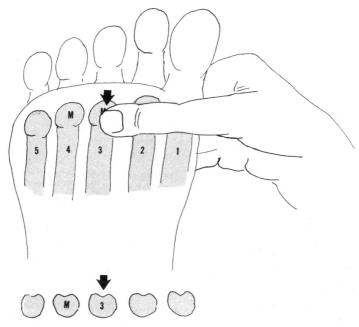

**Figure 5–32.** Diagnostic pressure site of metatarsalgia. Viewed from the plantar surface, digital pressure over the metatarsal head (M) is diagnostic of metatarsalgia. The precise site—(1), (2), (3), (4), or (5) metatarsal head—depends on the site of the pathology.

## Arthritis

In relation to the big toe, arthritis affects the first metatarsal-proximal-phalangeal joint, causing pain, crepitation, limited motion, and impaired gait,[8] because the big toe participates extensively in normal gait. A clinical examination includes an evaluation of the gait and determines at which stage of gait pain is experienced. Manually, the first metatarsophalangeal joint can be examined (see Fig. 5–26).

## Sesamoid Pain

Pain over the sesamoid bones is indicated by tenderness over them (see Fig. 5–25). There is often a callus.[9]

Morton's interdigital neuroma, which is discussed in Chapter 9, may confuse the examiner as to the exact site of pain near the metatarsal heads. Careful examination in which the head is digitally compressed, rather than the interdigital area, which contains the nerves, must be undergone (Fig. 5–34).

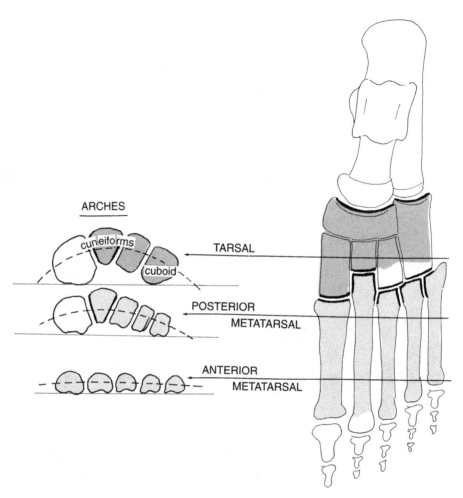

ARCHES

cuneiforms

cuboid

TARSAL

POSTERIOR
METATARSAL

ANTERIOR
METATARSAL

**Figure 5–33.** Muscular mechanism forming the transverse arch. The transverse arch is only a potentially flexible, not an anatomically structural arch. The metatarsal heads are raised by the toes with the toes kept straight and the metatarsophalangeal joints flexed (A) and (B) by the long and short flexors. Weakness of the intrinsic muscles permits the toes to flex at the interphalangeal joint, and the flexors then increase this flexion at the interphalangeal joints. The metatarsal heads thus bear the full body weight.

## MORTON'S SYNDROME: SHORT FIRST TOE

A short first metatarsal, termed *Morton's syndrome* (as described by Dudley Morton[10] not Thomas G. Morton,[11] who described metatarsalgia from a neuroma), causes excessive weight to be borne by the second metatarsal head. The condition is usually hereditary. It consists of the following: (1) an excessively short first metatarsal, which is hypermobile at its base where it articulates

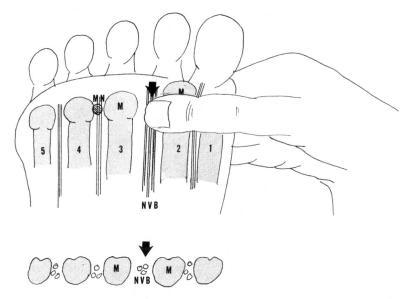

**Figure 5–34.** Diagnostic pressure site of interdigital neuroma. Viewed from the plantar surface, digital pressure over the neurovascular bundles (NVB), which form a neuroma between the metatarsal heads (M), is diagnostic of Morton's neuroma (MN). The precise site depends on the site of pathology and is usually between the third and fourth metatarsal heads, but various sites are possible.

with the second metatarsal and the cuneiform; (2) posterior displacement of the sesamoids; and (3) a thickening of the second metatarsal shaft (Fig. 5–35). The excessive weight borne by the second metatarsal causes excessive mobility at its base because of stress on the ligaments, capsules, and muscles that bind the second metatarsal with the cuneiform.

## MARCH FRACTURE

A march fracture is a stress fracture of a metatarsal bone, usually noted after a prolonged period of ambulation. A history of a violent injury is rare, making the initial diagnosis difficult since a "specific" traumatic activity is rarely determined.

The pathology is a hairline fracture of the shaft of the second or third metatarsal bone with no displacement of the fragments. Initially the fracture may not be noted on routine x-rays, but later, as callus forms about the fracture, a radiologic diagnosis is confirmed (Fig. 5–36). A bone scan will be diagnostic long before there is radiologic evidence.

Clinically, there is tenderness at the site of the fracture, and pain is noted by the patient on weight bearing and during flexion-extension of the toes of that

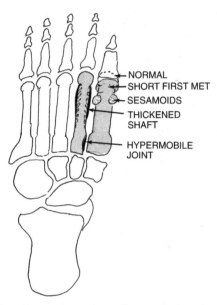

NORMAL
SHORT FIRST MET
SESAMOIDS
THICKENED
SHAFT
HYPERMOBILE
JOINT

**Figure 5–35.** The short first metatarsal: Dudley Morton syndrome. This syndrome of metatarsalgia consists of (1) a shorter than normal first metatarsal, (2) posterior displacement of the sesamoid bones, (3) excessive mobility of the first metatarsal at its base, and (4) thickening of the shaft of the second metatarsal caused by excessive weight bearing imposed on this bone. The resulting pain and tenderness are usually felt at the *base* of the first two metatarsals and the *head* of the second metatarsal.

phalanx. Pain subsides with rest and in the absence of weight bearing and recurs on resumption of weight bearing. Repeated weight bearing results in swelling and erythema at the fracture site.

## PES CAVUS

Pes cavus, also termed clawfoot or hollow foot, is a foot with an unusually high arch (Fig. 5–37). The high longitudinal arch causes a shortening of the foot and an obliquity of the metatarsal heads when they contact the floor surface. This may cause metatarsalgia and usually causes callus formation below the heads. The compensatory extension of the metatarsophalangeal joint causes a shortening of the extensor tendons with a tenodesis flexion of the proximal-middle phalangeal joint. The hyperflexed proximal-middle phalangeal joints cause callus formation at the dorsum of the toes. The metatarsophalangeal joints frequently dislocate, and the forefoot becomes inflexible.

Whether the cavus is anterior or posterior (Fig. 5–38) may be considered of academic interest but shows that degenerative changes of the talocalcaneal or

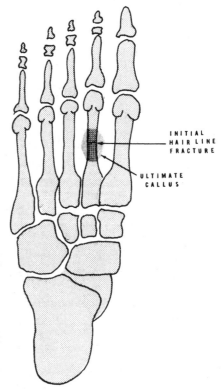

INITIAL
HAIR LINE
FRACTURE

ULTIMATE
CALLUS

**Figure 5–36.** March fracture of the second metatarsal. The initial fracture is often not observed during routine x-rays or may appear merely as a thin, hairline fracture. Within 3 weeks, after persistent pain, swelling, and tenderness, x-rays indicate bone callus formation. This may be the first positive radiologic diagnostic sign, but bone scans are positive at an earlier stage. Displacement of the bone fragments is rare.

forefoot joints may result. These changes ultimately are evident radiologically, but before significant organic changes occur, early joint pathology is evident on clinical examination.

Joint changes in the calcaneocuboid joint are palpable (Fig. 5–39). Changes in the cuboid–fifth metatarsal joint are also palpable (Figs. 5–40 and 5–41).

A high cavus foot may exist yet remain asymptomatic until calluses occur and/or articular changes become symptomatic. These articular changes may occur at the talocalcaneal or talar forefoot joints and can be elicited by appropriate manual testing. Gait may be impaired. Foot gear is usually difficult to acquire.

## TREATMENT PROTOCOLS

### Acute Foot Strain

Because acute foot strain is usually a self-limited condition that recovers on cessation of the activity, rest, elevation of the foot, use of oral salicylates or anti-

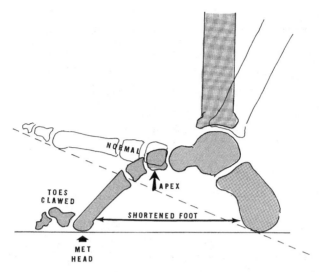

**Figure 5–37.** Pes cavus foot. The pes cavus foot has an exaggerated longitudinal arch with its apex at the naviculocuneiform joint. The foot is shorter than normal, the metatarsal heads are prominent, and the toes are clawed. This clawing is caused by contracture of the toe extensors. The distal phalanges are flexed, and there is a dislocation of the metatarsophalangeal joints. The dotted line placed horizontally depicts the weight-bearing normal foot and its longitudinal arch.

inflammatory medication, and local modalities such as ice or alternating ice and heat afford relief.

Evaluation of the foot and its mechanics may be indicated in the case where the activity postulated as the cause does not appear plausible and there is a functional impairment that can be prophylactically corrected.

## Chronic or Recurrent Foot Strain

In chronic or recurrent foot strain, symptomatic foot problems demand a careful evaluation of the foot structurally and functionally. Because the pronated foot is often the offender, this pronation must be corrected and the specific pathology addressed.

Initially, if the symptoms are severe and general foot rest allowing ambulation appears indicated, a soft (or hard) cast may be required. Molded, this cast allows the inflamed joints, tendons, ligaments, and muscles to recover. On removal of the cast and a careful evaluation, rehabilitation of the foot must be undertaken and the faulty mechanical aspects of the foot corrected. This is where the foot must be specifically evaluated and analyzed for causative factors. Prolonged immobilization is undesirable since disuse atrophy of all tissues occurs rapidly, aggravating the etiologic factors.

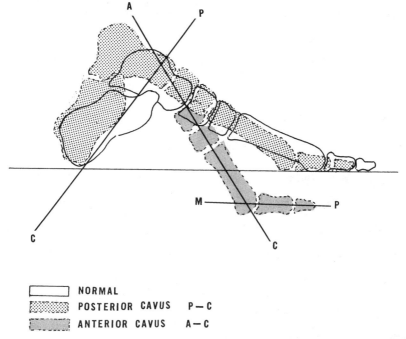

NORMAL
POSTERIOR CAVUS    P — C
ANTERIOR CAVUS    A — C

**Figure 5–38.** Cavus: Posterior or anterior. The normal foot's longitudinal arch is shown as the white foot. In posterior cavus (P-C), the hind foot is vertical with angulation at the talocalcaneal joint. In anterior cavus, the angulation is between the talus and the forefoot bones (A-C). Angulation is shown at the metatarsophalangeal joints (M-P).

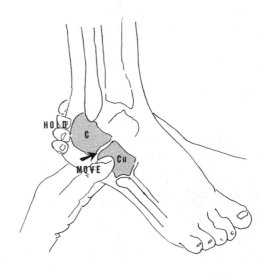

**Figure 5–39.** Palpation of the calcaneocuboid joint. Holding the calcaneus firmly (right hand), the cuboid can be mobilized with the left hand. This tests the mobility and pain production of a hypermobile calcaneocuboid joint.

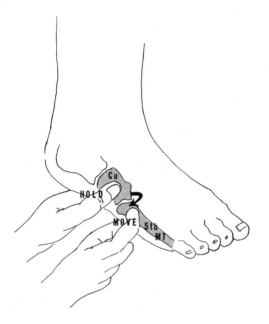

**Figure 5–40.** Palpation of the cuboid–fifth metatarsal joint. The flexibility and pain site of the cuboid–fifth metatarsal joint are tested by holding the cuboid (left hand) firmly and moving the fifth metatarsal bone (right hand).

Taping the foot into the desired shape is accepted as beneficial. Tape that includes adhesive-backed sponge rubber can alter the weight-bearing sites during stance and/or gait. The tape with sponge is cut in varying thicknesses, shapes, and sizes according to the desired ultimate function (Fig. 5–42). At best, this can only be considered a temporary remedy, since the pads must be replaced and modified frequently and are amenable to damage and alteration from wearing and wetting in showering and bathing.

Albeit that structural changes, osseous and articular, need to be corrected, when possible, exercises to increase flexibility and correct muscle imbalance should be considered early. Even if exercises are not corrective, per se, they enhance the recovery and augment the benefits of orthosis. Exercises benefit the ultimate success of surgery. In the event of any articular limitation or early contracture, the foot must be mobilized. This passive motion can be accomplished by a therapist, a relative, or even the patient. Specific exercises must be based on precise changes noted from the examination. Heel cord stretching exercises are standard. If they are indicated, they must be properly and repetitively performed (Fig. 5–43).

After the involved muscles are specifically identified, strengthening them must be addressed. Strengthening requires *active* exercises, with or without resistance, depending on the initial weakness or fatigability of the involved muscle. Circulation to the foot and lower leg is also enhanced by an active exercise program. Gait training and correction may also be valuable after the specific gait disorder is identified. Walking, if done properly and consistently, still remains the exercise of choice for total-body function. A cosmetic gait must be

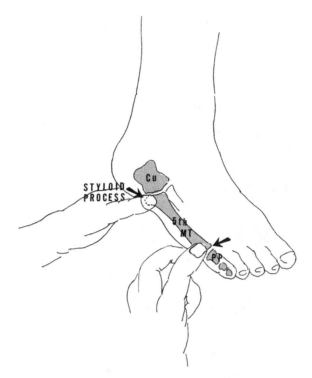

**Figure 5–41.** Palpation of the styloid process and the fifth metatarsophalangeal joint. The *upper hand* indicates palpation of the styloid process of the fifth metatarsal bone and, moving proximally, the cuboid metatarsal joint. The *lower hand* indicates the head of the fifth metatarsal, which articulates with the proximal phalanx (PP). If the lower hand mobilizes the fifth metatarsal, the upper hand can elicit motion, crepitation, and pain at the cuboid metatarsal joint.

assured as well as a therapeutic gait exercise program. Weight loss, if implicated, must be addressed.

Properly fitted *corrective* shoes must also be instituted. The term "corrective" is not an accurate concept, since shoes (Fig. 5–44), per se, do not correct: they merely allow the foot to function properly without constrictions or inhibitions. Examination of a well-worn shoe will often indicate the problems of gait (Fig. 5–45). If orthoses are indicated, shoes must be such as to allow the orthoses to be inserted, and the orthoses must be accepted by the patient. A properly fitted shoe can also maintain the alignment attempted by the orthosis.

Shoes should be fitted late in the day after prolonged ambulation since the normal foot "spreads" slightly and even deforms after a day's activities. The shoe should be broad across the forefoot and have a firm counter and a last that conforms to the gait style (Fig. 5–46). The shoe should be long enough to extend 1

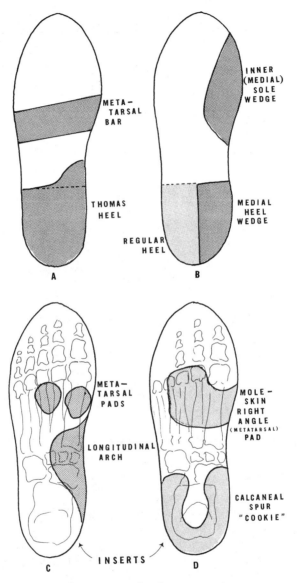

**Figure 5–42.** Shoe inserts and pads to minimize pressure sites.

inch past the big toe during weight bearing. The last should not be too firm or inflexible because some flexibility allows the intrinsic muscles of the foot to contract.

The heel should be reasonably narrow to minimize plantar flexion of the foot on stance. A high heel impairs the gait and ensures gliding forward of the foot during stance and gait, causing a forward movement into the narrower toe region.

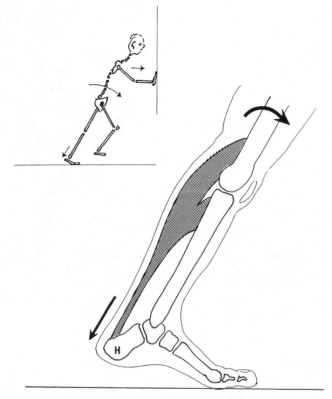

**Figure 5–43.** Heel cord stretching exercise. By leaning up against a wall and maintaining a heel-down position, the gastrocnemius-soleus muscle gets stretched. Going up and down makes the exercise active, as does bending the elbows. Starting farther from the wall increases the degree of stretch.

Appliances can be added to a shoe to assure the desired function. A heel addition such as a Thomas heel modifies the stance and the gait by altering the gait phases.

Orthoses that are molded to the foot to alter its shape have a valid place in foot strain correction. They must be molded to the weight-bearing foot and not impose any stress on any part of the foot, because discomfort will eliminate their being used. The orthoses must also be able to fit into a shoe and allow space for the foot after being inserted.

Ideally the foot should be casted and a positive mold made of the foot on which the orthosis is molded. The orthosis may be made of various materials such as a type of plastic, Plexiglas, and so on. Initially metal was used. Today metal may be used for reinforcement, but rarely is it the only material used.

The orthosis should include the heel to correct valgus or varus, which has been found to be a contributing factor in the disability. The forefoot pronation,

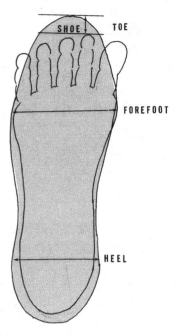

**Figure 5–44.** Proper fitting of shoes. The shoe toe should extend 1 inch ahead of the foot. At the forefoot, the shoe should be wide enough to allow the weight-bearing foot, at the end of a day of ambulation, to fit comfortably and not crowd the toes and metatarsal heads. The heel of the foot should be held snugly by the heel of the shoe.

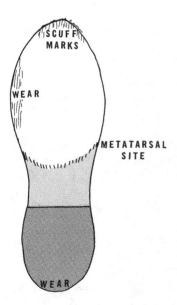

**Figure 5–45.** Examination of the sole of the shoe.

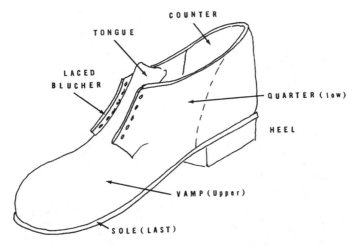

**Figure 5–46.** Components of the shoe.

which is usually the major pathology, is corrected and held by the orthosis. The longitudinal arch is also restored, as tolerated (Fig. 5–47).

The shoe heel may also be modified by wedging to control valgus or varus (Fig. 5–48). The heel must be held snugly to ensure that the wedge is effective (Fig. 5–49).

In the presence of metatarsalgia, pressure on the offending metatarsal heads may be eliminated by elevating the shafts of the specific metatarsal (Fig. 5–50). This pad must be under the shaft of the metatarsal and not under the

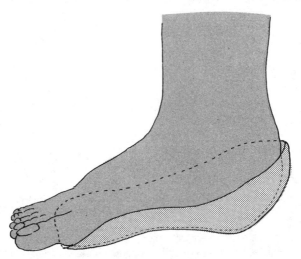

**Figure 5–47.** Molded orthotic device. The foot can be molded in the desired shape and supported by a molded plastic orthosis made from a plaster mold.

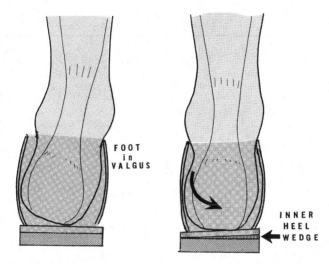

**Figure 5–48.** Ensuring a snug heel in controlling valgus or varus. *A* shows a valgus heel within a regular shoe with no correction. *B* shows an inner wedge in a shoe that is loose-fitting and thus does not correct the valgus. *C* indicates that inserting a corrective wedge within a close-fitted counter corrects the valgus.

head, because in that position, it would place additional pressure on the inflamed head. Because pronation is usually a factor in causing metatarsalgia, this must be addressed, including stretching the heel cord if this is found to be limited.

Calluses must be pared by soaking the foot in warm water and then using a stone or emory board. Preventing a recurrence of callus must include assess-

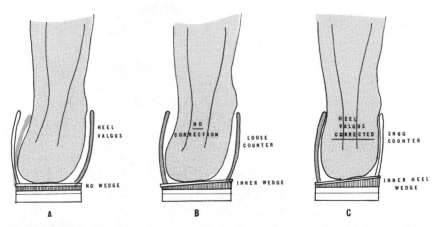

**Figure 5–49.** Inner heel wedge to treat heel valgus. An inner wedge should taper from no elevation at the outer border to 1/16 to 3/16 inches on the inner border. The exact elevation is determined by the height needed to place the calcaneus in a vertical position.

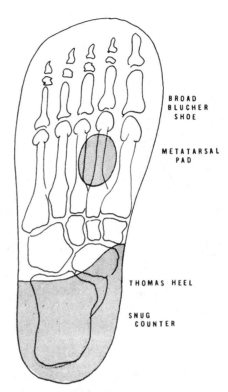

BROAD
BLUCHER
SHOE

METATARSAL
PAD

THOMAS HEEL

SNUG
COUNTER

**Figure 5–50.** Shoe modifications in treatment of metatarsalgia. A pad placed behind the second metatarsal head elevates the shaft and diminishes the weight-bearing on the offending metatarsal head. The broad forefoot shoe with a soft upper permits the foot to spread without cramping or constriction. A Thomas heel assists in correcting pronation during gait. A snug counter assures a central heel.

ing the cause of callus formation. Padding around and under the lesion should be instituted while the normal biomechanics of the foot are restored.[12,13]

A full-length weight-bearing insert with varying thickness is molded to the foot (Fig. 5–51). The insert is thicker just proximal to the offending metatarsal head and is hollowed out under the painful callus. The insert is covered with a soft-grade polyethylene foam (Plastazote*) and is thickened using cork or multiple layers of the insert material. The hollowed-out areas are filled with a viscoelastic polymer to retard "bottoming out."

Surgically, the offending calluses may be pared by a scalpel used by a physician, trained nurse, or trained technician. A powered surgical sander is used[†] to literally sand down the callus.

Treatment of big toe pathology, discussed in Chapter 6, must conform to a general concept. Because the toe extends and flexes repeatedly during each phase of gait, it is a common cause of pain and impairment when its mobility is impaired. The toe and its first metatarsal must also be in direct alignment, which is not true in many painful hallux problems.

---

*Plastazote, Apex Foot Health, South Hackensack, New Jersey.

[†]Dremel, Division of Emerson Electrical Company, Racine, Wisconsin.

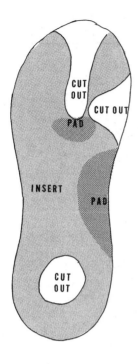

**Figure 5–51.** Multilayered sole insert used in treatment of calluses. A precisely cut out insert that fits into the shoe is made of polyethylene material of varying thickness. Where indicated, there are cutouts over the offending callus. Padding made by increasing the thickness of the polyethylene and/or insertion of cork further minimizes pressure on the callus or the offending bone.

To prevent extension of the sole of the shoe when there is limited hallux motion, a steel shank may be inserted within the outer and inner midsole of the shoe (Fig. 5–52). A *rocker sole* is also effective in conditions of painfully limited motion of the metatarsal first phalanx of the hallus (Fig. 5–53).

Sesamoid problems are best treated by minimizing direct trauma. Because the sesamoids are contained within the tendons, their movement combined with compression against the metatarsal head must be minimized or avoided. A provocative test is reproduction of the pain by passive hyperextension of the toe with reproduction of the pain at the exact site of the sesamoid. The steel shank (see Fig. 5–52) and the rocker sole (see Fig. 5–53) are indicated. Before resorting to surgical resection, a time factor must be allowed. Transcutaneous electrical nerve stimulation (TENS)[4] has been effective.

Hyperextension of the toes, which causes excessive exposure of the metatarsal heads and a "clawing" of the toes as they compensatorily flex, may be surgically treated by extensor tenotomy and/or capsulotomy of the metatarsophalangeal joint. Resection of the distal phalangeal heads may be needed. Such surgical intervention is beyond the scope of this text and is best referred to a specialized orthopedic surgeon.

Treatment of Morton's syndrome requires building a "platform" under the first metatarsal to relieve the weight bearing on the second metatarsal.

In a march fracture, rest, elevation, anti-inflammatory medication, and modalities of ice or alternate ice and heat are initially effective. A short plaster

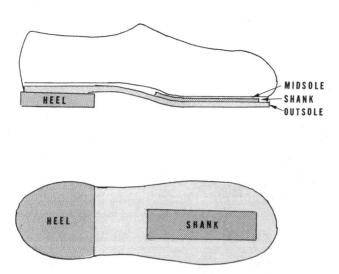

**Figure 5–52.** Steel shank insert. Where there is evidence that the hyperextension of the phalanges is contributing to anterior foot pain, the sole of the shoe can be made inflexible by inserting a steel shank between the midsole and outer sole. This prevents extension of the toes during the late stance phase and heel-off.

cast may be needed to allow ambulation during healing. As there is no bony displacement, no further care is needed unless it becomes evident that a foot problem may have contributed to the march fracture.

Cavus foot, with symptomatic metarsalgia and/or degenerative changes in the forefoot, is best treated by a laminated insert using cork and a superficial layer of Plastazote. The metatarsal heads are protected by cutouts filled with viscoelastic polyester (Fig. 5–51).

Conservative care of foot problems obviously demands a careful pathoanatomic kinetic evaluation of the foot that addresses all aspects of shoe corrections, orthosis, inserts,[14,15] and possible surgical intervention when all conservative approaches fail to afford the needed result.

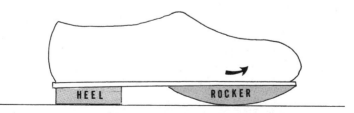

**Figure 5–53.** Rocker sole. Applying a rocker sole to the shoe allows the foot to pass through mid- and last stance phases and heel-off without extending the sole and thus extending the toes during these phases of gait.

# REFERENCES

1. Cailliet, R: Soft Tissue Pain and Disability, ed 3. FA Davis, Philadelphia, 1996.
2. Clayton, LT (ed): Taber's Cyclopedic Medical Dictionary, ed 17. FA Davis, Philadelphia, 1993, pp 1733, 1760.
3. Tillman, LJ, and Cummings, GS: Biological Mechanisms of Connective Tissue Mutability, Chap 1. In Currier, DP, and Nelson, RM: Dynamics of Human Biological Tissues. FA Davis, Philadelphia, 1992, pp 1–44.
4. Cailliet, R: Pain: Mechanisms and Management. FA Davis, Philadelphia, 1993.
5. Sjolander, P, Djupsjpbacka, M, Johansson, H, Sojka, P, and Lorentzon, R: Can receptors in the collateral ligaments contribute to knee joint stability and proprioception via effects on the fusiform–muscle spindle system? Neuro-Orthopedics 15:65–80, 1994.
6. Hall, MG, Ferrell, WR, Baxendale, RH, and Hamblen, DL: Knee Joint Proprioception: Threshold Detection Levels in Healthy Young Subjects. Neuro-Orthopedics 15:81–90, 1994.
7. Gould, JS: Metatarsalgia. Orthop Clin North Am 20(4):553–562, 1989.
8. Thompson, FM, and Mann, RA: Arthritides. In Mann, RA (ed): Surgery of the Foot, ed 5. CV Mosby, St. Louis, 1986, p 158.
9. Mann, RA: Keratotic disorders of the plantar skin. In Mann, RA (ed): Surgery of the Foot, ed 5. CV Mosby, St. Louis, 1986, p 192.
10. Morton, DJ: The Human Foot. Columbia University Press, New York, 1948.
11. Morton, TG: Interdigital neuroma. Am J Med Sci 71:37, 1876.
12. Reynolds, JC: Metatarsalgia. In Gould, JS (ed): The Foot Book. Williams & Wilkins, Baltimore, 1988.
13. Smith, RW: Calluses: Nonsurgical treatment: In Gould, JS (ed): The Foot Book. Williams & Wilkins, Baltimore, 1988.
14. Zamosky, I, and Licht, S: Shoes and Their Modifications. In Licht, S (ed): Orthotics Etcetera: Physical Medicine Library, Vol 9. Elizabeth Licht, Publisher, New Haven, 1966.
15. Milgram, JE: Office measures for relief of the painful foot. J Bone Joint Surg 46-A:1096, 1964.

# CHAPTER 6

# The Great Toe

The great toe provides stability for the medial aspect of the foot[1] through the windlass mechanism of the plantar aponeurosis (Fig. 6–1).[2] The plantar aponeurosis arises from the tubercle of the calcaneus and passes forward to insert into the bases of the proximal phalanges. During gait as the body passes over the foot, the big toe, being in the neutral position, dorsiflexes as the heel rises off the floor. It then plantar flexes prior to toe-off (Figs. 6–2 and 6–3).

Force plate analysis demonstrates that there is increased pressure under the first metatarsal head that transfers to the first hallux in the second half of the stance phase as the gait enters the toe-off phase.[3]

## HALLUX VALGUS

As stated in Chapter 2, the "normal" foot must be pain-free and have normal muscle balance, an absence of contracture, a central heel, straight and mobile toes, and three sites of weight bearing while standing and during the stance phase of walking.[4]

*Hallux valgus* is a static subluxation of the first metatarsophalangeal joint. There are three components of the *bunion complex*: (1) the large toe angulates laterally toward the second toe, (2) the medial portion of the first metatarsal head enlarges, and (3) the bursa over the medial aspect of the metatarsophalangeal joint becomes inflamed and thick walled (Fig. 6–3). This condition is most frequently found in older women who have a broadened forefoot with a flattened transverse arch in a pronated foot. The big toe frequently displaces the second toe. Although most frequently first noted in elderly women, this condition will have been present in the patient since early life. However, the condition only becomes symptomatic when the inflamed tissues become painful. Hallux valgus

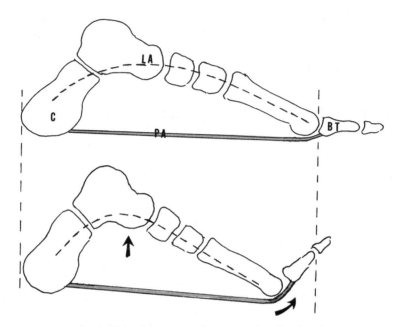

**Figure 6–1.** Windlass effect of big toe on longitudinal arch. The plantar aponeurosis (PA) attaches to the calcaneus (C) and the proximal phalanx of the big toe (BT). The normal longitudinal arch (LA) is shown in the top figure. In the bottom figure, as the toe extends (curved arrow), the plantar aponeurosis curves around the big toe and elevates the longitudinal arch (vertical arrow).

occurs almost exclusively in people who wear inappropriate shoes,[5] although it does sometimes develop in people who wear modest, proper footwear.

If there is a variance in the alignment of the first hallux, the stabilization mechanism of the big toe is diminished because the windlass effect is lessened. This results in a lateral transfer of weight bearing to the second and even the third metatarsal.

Because surgical intervention in abnormalities may interfere with the windlass mechanism, this change in the mechanism must be understood. Intervention such as the Keller procedure, which removes the base of the proximal phalanx, destroys the windlass mechanism and transfers the weight to the second metatarsal head. Any osteotomy that shortens the metatarsal more than 7 to 10 mm results in decreased weight bearing and thus transfers the weight laterally.

The metatarsophalangeal joint of the first toe differs from the other toes in that it has a sesamoid mechanism. The head of the first metatarsal has a cartilage-covered ovoid head that articulates with a smaller, concave, elliptically shaped base of the proximal phalanx (Fig. 6–4).

Fan-shaped ligamentous bands join the collateral ligaments of the metatarsophalangeal joint. The ligament runs distally and in a plantar direction to

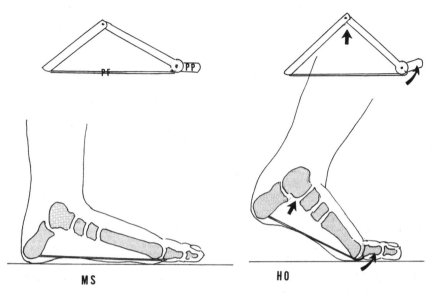

**Figure 6–2.** Plantar fascia windlass effect upon proximal phalanx. At midstance phase of gait (MS), the proximal phalanx (PP) is in a neutral position. As gait progresses to heel-off (HO), the longitudinal arch angle increases (arrow) and the plantar fascia wraps around the head of the metatarsal and the big toe extends (curved arrow). A reflex flexor muscle reaction causes the big toe to ultimately flex and plantar-press to the floor.

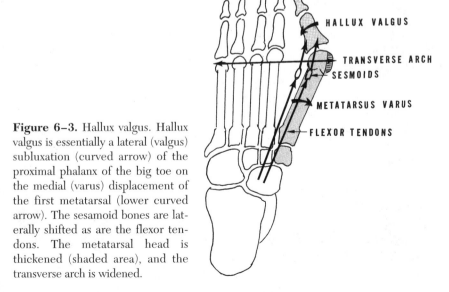

**Figure 6–3.** Hallux valgus. Hallux valgus is essentially a lateral (valgus) subluxation (curved arrow) of the proximal phalanx of the big toe on the medial (varus) displacement of the first metatarsal (lower curved arrow). The sesamoid bones are laterally shifted as are the flexor tendons. The metatarsal head is thickened (shaded area), and the transverse arch is widened.

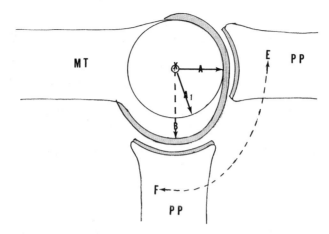

**Figure 6–4.** Metatarsophalangeal joint of hallux. The lateral view of the metatarsophalangeal joint of the hallux reveals covering by cartilage (dark area) with the metatarsal head being ovoid (B > A) rather than round ($A_1$). The base of the proximal phalanx (PP) is more rounded and smaller in surface. In full flexion (F), the distance from the axis (X) is greater in full flexion than in full extension (E), indicating this joint to be incongruous.

attach to the proximal phalanx, and the *fan* moves in a plantar direction to attach to the sesamoids and the plantar pads.

On the plantar surface of the metatarsal head are two parallel grooves. The sesamoid bones contained within the flexor hallucis brevis tendons are convex and "ride" within these grooves. The sesamoids are attached to the base of the phalanx and *not* to the metatarsal head. This means that the sesamoids move in whatever direction the great toe moves (Fig. 6–5).

The first metatarsal head has no muscle inserting on it and is thus supported by a capsular sling. In a hallux valgus, when the metatarsal moves laterally and the proximal phalanx medially, the extensor hallucis longus and the flexor hallucis longus deviate their force laterally, accentuating the deforming forces. The sesamoid bones also migrate and the fibular sesamoid becomes uncovered, allowing the abductor hallucis muscle to slide under the metatarsal head, causing pronation of the great toe.

The only structure that affords medial stability of the metatarsophalangeal joint is the medial ligamentous complex, which fails when the etiologic forces are imposed.

## Etiologic Concepts

In ordinary orthopedic practice, hallux valgus is seen more frequently in adults. Yet with careful questioning, many, if not most, patients recall deformity occurring in early life.[6,7] Many concepts have been proposed regarding the eti-

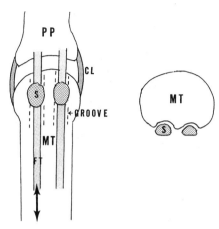

**Figure 6–5.** Sesamoid paths along metatarsal head. There are grooves in the plantar aspect of the metatarsal head (MT) in which the flexor tendons (FT) glide (arrows). The sesamoids (S) are enclosed within the tendon that attaches to the base of the proximal phalanx (PP). The capsules (CL) of the M-P joint are shown.

ology of hallux valgus. Congenital factors may, and probably do, predispose to deformity in later life.

The first metatarsal may be shorter than normal and may be in varus as a residue of congenital metatarsus primus varus (see Fig. 4–18). Review of English orthopedic literature implies that metatarsus varus is the underlying cause of hallux valgus, but there is little evidence that this is a valid claim.[6,7]

Whether the lateral deviation of the proximal phalanx occurs first rather than secondary to primary metatarsus varus remains unproved. This remains a bone of contention since permanent correction of the condition (hallux valgus) cannot be expected unless the "primary" condition has been corrected.[8,9]

The intermetatarsal angle increases (normally) with age and thus, along with other forces, can increase the incidence of hallux valgus. Subluxation of the first metatarsophalangeal joint occurs frequently before the epiphysis is closed, implying a "young" incidence of hallux valgus.[6,10]

The varus of the first metatarsal may be brought about by the obliquity of the first cuneiform bone, which changes the angle of the first metatarsal joint (Fig. 6–6A). The head of the first metatarsal may be more convex than normal and may permit the first proximal phalanx to shift laterally (Fig. 6–6B). Primary or secondary muscular imbalance will pull the first phalanx laterally and overcome an ineffectual abductor hallucis (Fig. 6–6C).

Repeated trauma from wearing narrow, pointed shoes and/or high heels, uncorrected pronation, added weight, and debilitated intrinsic muscles allow the big toe to deviate progressively in a lateral direction. The long tendons, both flexor and extensor, of the big toe (see Fig. 6–5) shift laterally along with their enclosed sesamoid bones and exert traction, causing further valgus (Fig. 6–6B). The adductor hallucis tendon is a relatively fixed structure, which inserts into the base of the proximal phalanx and thus simultaneously anchors the sesamoids so they cannot drift medially with the metatarsal head.

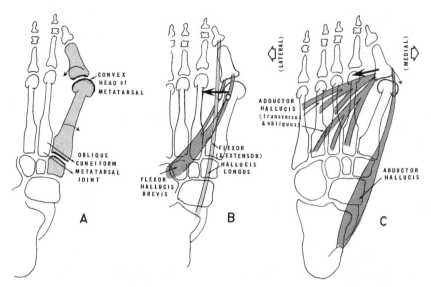

**Figure 6–6.** Concepts of etiology of hallux valgus. The most probable causes held responsible for hallux valgus are shown in the following parts. (*A*) Excessive convexity of the head of the first metatarsal, permitting the proximal phalanx to sublux laterally. There is also an oblique articular surface of the cuneiform that causes the metatarsal to deviate in a varus direction. (*B*) As the phalanx deviates laterally, the flexor hallucis brevis and longus tendons on the plantar foot surface and the extensor hallucis longus tendon on the dorsum of the foot migrate laterally and act as a bowstring force. (*C*) Imbalance of the foot intrinsics causes the adductors to overpull and shorten, overpowering the abductors, which then elongate.

As valgus of the hallux occurs, the base of the proximal phalanx pushes the metatarsal head medially. This attenuates the medial capsule. The abductor hallucis, which inserts on the medial aspect of the proximal phalanx, moves medially. The cartilage of the metatarsal head gradually smooths out and no longer becomes resistant to this migration (Fig. 6–7).

Whether there is rotation of the metatarsal shaft, which has been postulated,[11] is questioned. If there is some pronation of the foot, the great toe undergoes longitudinal rotation, placing the relationship of the metatarsophalangeal joint at an oblique position to the floor. This places the joint at a mechanical disadvantage regarding the force applied to the joint in everyday activities. Many surgeons feel that failure of surgical procedures is brought about by a failure to correct this rotation.

## Bunions

Many patients present to physicians for hallux valgus because of the presence of a "bunion," which is cosmetically unacceptable, causes pain, and prevents acquiring affordable, acceptable footwear.

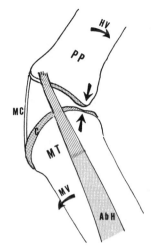

**Figure 6–7.** Mechanism of hallux valgus. Valgus motion of the hallux (HV) causes the lateral aspect of the proximal phalanx (PP) to impinge (straight arrows) upon the opposing cartilage (C) of the metatarsal head (MT). On further wear, there is thinning of the cartilage, which decreases resistance to further motion. The medial capsule (MC) becomes stretched and the tendon of the abductor hallucis (AbH) migrates laterally, adding another valgus force.

A bony outgrowth of the metatarsophalangeal is not noted early in hallux valgus. What appears as a prominence is a displacement of the proximal phalanx in a lateral direction. As the condition progresses, the phalanx deviates further in a lateral direction, and the sagittal groove on the head of the medial metatarsal head deepens as the medial eminence proliferates. The sagittal groove (see Fig. 6–6) migrates laterally as do the flexor tendon and its sesamoid, both of which thicken. Both gradually become attenuated as they are mechanically inefficient.

The overlying bursa on the medial aspect of the joint becomes inflamed, gradually thickens, and ultimately calcifies (Fig. 6–8). As the ligament of the medial sesamoid thickens, so does the medial collateral ligament, which gradually becomes attenuated because there is external friction.

## Muscular Action in Hallux Valgus

The muscular dynamics of the formation of the hallux valgus can be understood by evaluating their function. The long and short extensor tendons pass dorsally, and the long and short flexors pass on the plantar surface. The conjoined tendons of the abductor and adductor hallucis pass medially and laterally, respectively.

The joint capsule is covered only by the hood ligaments, which hold the extensor hallucis longus tendon in place. As valgus motion develops, the medial hood capsule and the ligaments elongate, allowing the extensor hallucis longus tendon to migrate and contract. It now no longer merely extends the hallux but also adducts it. As shown in Figure 6–7, the abductor hallucis also becomes a deforming factor.

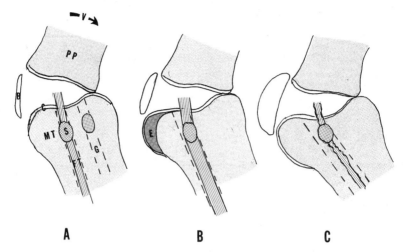

**Figure 6–8.** Formation of a "bunion." Part *A* depicts the prebunion hallux valgus (V). The bursa (B) is normal, as is the cartilage (C). The sesamoid bones (S) within the flexor tendons (FT) are within normal grooves (G) on the plantar surface of the metatarsal heads (MT). The articulation with the proximal phalanx (PP) shows its angulation. Part *B* is the stage of bunion development where there is thickening (exostosis E) of the medial aspect of the metatarsal head. The bursa thickens and the grooves widen. The flexor tendons thicken. Part *C* is a later stage, where the bunion is now well established and the bursa large and thickened. The flexor tendons are frayed.

In 15% to 20% of patients with hallux valgus, a dislocation of the second toe occurs. The second toe has two dorsal and two plantar interossei (see Fig. 1–29). Their tendons extend either dorsolaterally or dorsomedially, depending on the alignment of the phalanges. With the metatarsophalangeal joint in direct alignment, they act either as adductor or as abductor. As the metatarsophalangeal joint extends the base of the proximal phalanx, it is pulled dorsally by these muscles.

If the foot is kept in a constant, toe-extended position, such as wearing a high heel does, the plantar capsule becomes overstretched. With valgus of the hallux, the big toe veering laterally moves under the second toe and gradually dislocates it (Fig. 6–9).

## Examination

Evaluation of the patient with hallux valgus (frequently the complaint is of a painful "bunion") is to ascertain the main complaint. It may merely be that the broad forefoot makes wearing normal shoes impossible. Or there may be pain

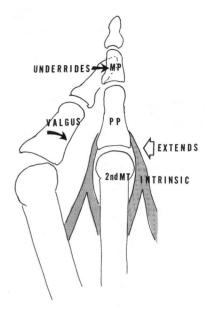

**Figure 6–9.** Mechanism of dislocation of second toe from hallux valgus. The intrinsics of the metatarsal can become extensors of the proximal phalanx if the toes are kept in chronic extension, such as occurs from wearing high heels. The phalanges of the hallux (first toe) migrate laterally under the elevated second toes and gradually dislocate them.

on movement of the big toe, rubbing of the second toe, which has been dorsally displaced by the valgus of the hallux, or a painful swelling of the medial aspect of the first metatarsophalangeal joint.

Examination of the standing, barefoot patient accentuates the weight-bearing foot and its deformities (Fig. 6–10). In the seated position, the foot is actively moved at all joints, and the movement of the first metatarsophalangeal and distal phalangeal joints can be observed. Limitation, crepitation, and even production of pain become apparent. Passive range of motion of each joint is then performed. Degree of mobility is noted as being limited or hypermobile. Callus formations are also noted.

## Radiologic Studies

Radiologic studies are then performed in a weight-bearing position and include anterior-posterior, lateral, and oblique views. The following must be analyzed:

- The angle of the valgus of the hallux
- The intermetatarsal angle
- The degree of the hallux interphalangeus
- The size of the medial eminence
- Evidence of degenerative changes in the first metatarsophalangeal joint
- Obliquity of the first metatarsocuneiform joint
- The presence of a lateral facet at the base of the first metatarsal shaft
- Determination of the congruity of the metatarsophalangeal joint[12]

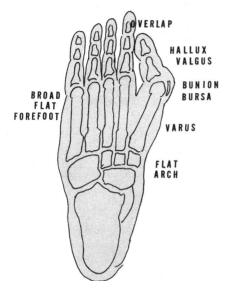

BROAD
FLAT
FOREFOOT

OVERLAP

HALLUX
VALGUS

BUNION
BURSA

VARUS

FLAT
ARCH

**Figure 6–10.** The foot with hallux valgus and bunion. The foot with hallux valgus has a broad forefoot, a depressed metartarsal, and longitudinal arches. Often the hallux overrides the second toe, which may become a hammer toe with callus. A swollen, tender bursa may override the enlarged medial aspect of the first metatarsal head.

The following angles must be measured (Fig. 6–11). The hallux valgus angle is formed by a line that passes through the proximal phalanx, forming an angle with a line drawn through the first metatarsal. The angle (HV in Fig. 6–11) is essentially the angle of deviation from direct alignment of the hallux with the metatarsal. Up to 10° is considered normal, with an angle of 15° considered abnormal.[12] The intermetatarsal angle (IM) measures the relationship of the first metatarsal bone to the second and depicts the degree of metatarsus varus.

There may be malalignment of the metatarsophalangeal joint, which is usually not associated with arthrosis. When present, degenerative changes must be ascertained. This is done clinically by finding painful limitation and/or crepitation and is confirmed radiologically.

The size of an enlarged medial eminence ("bunion") must be determined and ascertained clinically as being the concern. A large HV angle may also implicate instability of the joint, which must be determined clinically, not radiologically.

An enlarged lateral facet at the base of the first metatarsal may block realignment of the first metatarsal and mandate an osteotomy if clinically significant. The congruity of the metatarsocuneiform joint must also be ascertained as to being a factor in the production of symptomatic hallux valgus. Absence of lateral subluxation speaks against incongruity in spite of there being a hallux valgus. Lateral subluxation indicates incongruity, which further indicates that correction can be accomplished by "sliding" the proximal phalanx into an anatomic alignment.

It is apparent from the above that the decision as to the type and extent of hallux valgus and its correction demands determining the proper patho-

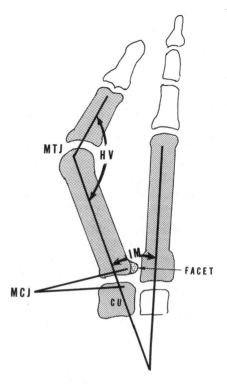

**Figure 6-11.** Hallux valgus angle. Radiologically the following angles can be measured: HV = hallux valgus angle (should be less than 15°); IM = inter-metatarsal angle (should be less than 9°); MCJ = metatarsocuneiform angle; MTJ = metatarsophalangeal joint (to reveal degenerative changes).

anatomic basis for the condition. Patient expectations from any corrective procedure must also be clarified because none will create a "new foot" or necessarily a pain-free one that permits wearing any type of shoe. Mere anatomic realignment is not an assurance. Even a mild deformity may result in some stiffness, joint pain, joint limitation, and even some nerve entrapment.

Shoe wear must be carefully addressed because wearing narrow-toe-box shoes and high heels will undoubtedly never be acceptable. Even successful surgical anatomic correction will not allow wearing inappropriate shoes, even if they are socially desirable.

## Treatment

Treatment must be individualized according to the age of the patient, the degree of deformity, the severity and duration of the symptoms, and the definite relationship of the symptoms to the hallux valgus. Many persons with severe deformity are pain-free and not disabled. Cosmetic concern especially deserves guarded diagnosis and treatment.

A person who develops hallux valgus before the age of 20 and who has a family history should be treated conservatively and prophylactically. Proper shoe wear that corrects or modifies the pes planus and foot pronation must be addressed. A broad-forefoot shoe must be stressed. A stabilizing splint should be worn at night (Fig. 6–12). The shoe should have a flat heel, and a pouch may be punched out or cut out over the bunion and bursa. In the elderly, molded shoes that prevent pressure on the bunion and bursa are effective. Correction of the pronation, as tolerated, must be instituted as well as correction of the flattened longitudinal arch. Exercises have their advocates but are of a questionable value.

A full discussion of surgical interventions is beyond the scope of this text because these are numerous and varied. However, general principles can be discussed.

Osteotomy of the proximal phalanx, combined with excision of the medial exostosis, is a standard procedure (Fig. 6–13). Distal soft-tissue procedures that release the contracted tissues are also common. Numerous procedures include proximal osteotomy of the metatarsal, which does not shorten the length of the metatarsal bone, and hence does not alter the windlass effect, which can prevent functional first phalanx dorsiflexion and plantar flexion.

With a hypermobile first metatarsocuneiform joint, an arthrodesis has its advocates. When there are severe degenerative changes in the metatarsophalangeal joint, an arthrodesis is also contemplated.[13,14]

A recent tricorrectional bunionectomy has been proposed that appears physiologically sound[15] because it prevents shortening and elevation of the involved metatarsal.

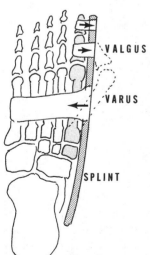

**Figure 6–12.** Night splint for juvenile hallux valgus. In a forefoot that has flexibility and can be manually corrected, a night splint that adducts the first metatarsal (corrects the varus) and abducts the two phalanges (corrects the valgus) is effective.

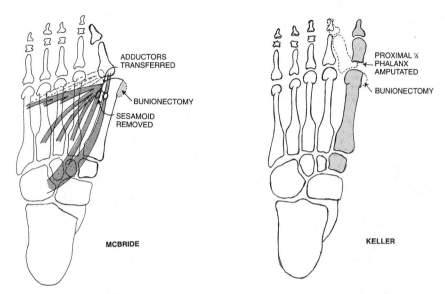

**Figure 6–13.** Surgical procedures for correcting hallux valgus. The *McBride* procedure consists of trimming the bunion, plicating the capsule on the medial aspect of the metatarsal head, and transplanting the adductor conjoined tendon from the base of the proximal phalanx to the outer head of the metatarsal. The adductor group now pulls the metatarsal laterally and does not sublux the phalanx The *Keller* procedure trims the bunion and amputates the proximal third of the proximal phalanx. The muscular attachments to the phalanx are removed, allowing the sesamoids to retract and the big toe to shorten.

In summary, decisions are based on the following:

1. The congruity of the metatarsophalangeal joint.
2. The degree of valgus greater than 15°.
3. The presence of degenerative symptomatic changes in either the metatarsophalangeal or metatarsocuneiform joints.

Presurgical evaluation may also be followed postsurgically by electromyographic analysis studies as well as clinical observations and patient satisfaction.

With or without surgical intervention, the individual with the hallus valgus foot will probably not be able to wear "standard shoes" and shoes will need modification (Fig. 6–14).

## Electromyographic Analysis Studies

Besides using foot pressure mapping to evaluate gait abnormalities (see Chap. 2), electromyographic studies are also being pursued. These studies have been extensively used in laboratory settings but are now having clinical application. When synchronized with mapping, they provide valuable information that should be considered before beginning any surgical intervention.

Six superficial skin electrodes are placed over the muscle bellies of the right and left tibialis anterior, peroneus longus, and medial gastrocnemius. The precise location is determined by having the patient perform a 5-second isometric contraction.

During gait and employing pressure mapping, the EMG is synchronized and recorded with the pressure mapping. The peroneus longus muscle controls the first metatarsal against the ground reaction forces. One of the major causes of bunion deformity is an elevation of the first metatarsal, which is called *hypermobility of the first ray*.[16] This allegedly contributes to formation of the bunion and limiting the motion of the hallux.

Generally, the peroneus longus and the extensor propulsion forces are dysfunctional when hallux valgus deformity develops in the pronated foot. Now, besides examining the patient with hallux valgus in the seated position, ambula-

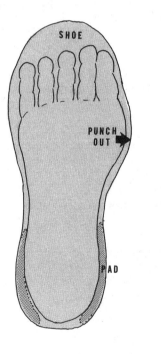
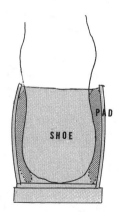

**Figure 6–14.** Shoe modification in hallux valgus bunion. In hallux valgus with bunion, the forefoot is excessively broad and the protruding bunion presents a specific problem. The forefoot aspect of the shoe can be "punched out." Because a broad-forefoot shoe may also have a broad heel counter, pads may be inserted to make the heel snug.

tory testing is possible. Mapping and concomitant EMG studies now record the exact mechanics of the patient's gait, which cannot be accurately evaluated by the human eye.

## HALLUX RIGIDUS

Hallux rigidus is the second most common painful problem of the big toe. The metatarsophalangeal joint of the hallux (big toe) dorsiflexes and plantar flexes repeatedly during gait. Thus, when this joint loses its flexibility, gait is impaired. Pain occurs when there are secondary degenerative changes of the cartilage, causing degenerative arthrosis. As the foot passes over from the mid-stance phase, it dorsiflexes and the big toe extends.

Since there is push-off of the foot, the big toe plantar flexes. The tendons of the flexor muscles contain the sesamoid bones, which further contribute to the mechanism and thus the pathology when the cartilage undergoes degeneration. Degenerative changes undergo various stages from merely softening of the cartilage with some synovitis to significant degeneration with partial fusion. This is discussed in Chapter 5.

Pain is noted at every step. The patient excessively supinates the weight-bearing foot in an attempt to place the weight to the outer border of the foot and avoid motion at the first ray, the inner border. During gait, the weight "rolls off" the fifth metatarsal head. Fatigue occurs as the gait is significantly impaired and the foot gradually acquires calluses on the parts bearing weight (fifth metatarsal head), and the joints of the fifth metatarsal and proximal phalanx may undergo early degeneration.

### Diagnosis

The diagnosis is made by the patient indicating "when" during gait the pain occurs and "where" the pain is felt. The examination of the first metatarsophalangeal joint (see Figs. 5–26 and 5–27) reveals crepitation, limited painful range of motion, and deformity of the joint. The sesamoid bones can also be palpated (see Fig. 5–25) and cause pain as well as being painful on forceful extension of the hallux. Radiologic studies reveal the extent of articular damage.

### Treatment

Prevention of motion of the first metatarsal proximal phalanx during gait is indicated. This is accomplished by the use of a steel shank in the shoe (see Fig.

5–52) or the use of a rocker sole (see Fig. 5–53) (Fig. 6–15). A pad insert placed under the shaft of the first metatarsal raises the bone and decreases the degree of flexion of the metatarsophalangeal joint.

In early degenerative changes where there is some motion, even though it is painful and limited, conservative measures usually suffice. Interarticular injection of an analgesic agent with or without steroids gives temporary relief. Oral anti-inflammatory medications afford some relief. Because joint motion gradually decreases until there is total fusion, surgical intervention is elective.

Once the joint is fused, articular changes occur at more proximal joints of the first metatarsal, and callus formation occurs at the pressure sites upon the first toe.

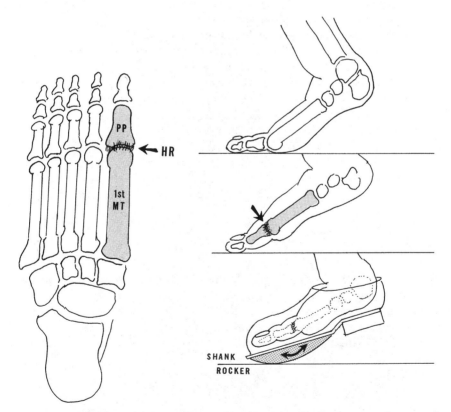

**Figure 6–15.** Hallux rigidus. In a damaged joint between the first metatarsal (MT) and the proximal phalanx (PP), the joint does not move or does so painfully at every step (*upper* figure on the right). Treatment is to prevent dorsiflexion of the big toe at each step, which is accomplished by inserting a steel shank in the shoe, preventing flexion of the sole, and placing a rocker bottom to the sole. This permits a pain-free gait.

## HAMMER TOES

A hammer toe is a fixed-flexion deformity of the interphalangeal joints (between the metatarsal and proximal phalanx and the proximal and middle phalanges). The distal phalanx also usually flexes but is not fixed and may point straight ahead.

Calluses form on the dorsum of the flexed interphalangeal joints (Fig. 6–16). The proximal phalanx will often sublux from the capsule being over-stretched, and the capsules and tendons on the flexed (plantar surfaces) side will contract. If the flexion deformity is mainly or exclusively in the distal joint, the condition is termed a *mallet toe*.

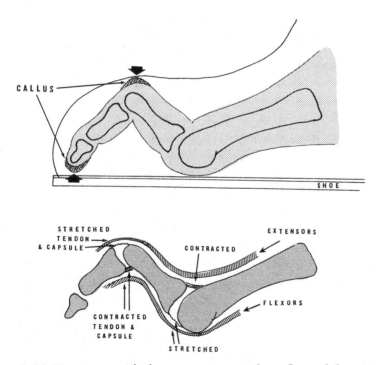

**Figure 6–16.** Hammer toes. The hammer toe is most often a flexion deformity of the interphalangeal joint, usually in the second, third, and fourth toes. The capsules on the concave side shorten (contract), and those on the extensor side hyperextend. Subluxation occurs frequently. Although the proximal and middle phalangeal joint is flexed, the prox-imal phalanx is extended. The distal phalanx may be either flexed or extended. Calluses occur at the dorsal surface of the proximal phalanx and may occur at the tip of the distal phalanx (arrows).

# REFERENCES

1. Mann, RA: The great toe. Orthop Clin North Am 20(4):519–533, 1989.
2. Hicks, JH: The mechanism of the foot. II. The plantar aponeurosis and the arch. J Anat 88:25, 1954.
3. Clark, TE: The pressure distribution under the foot during barefoot walking (dissertation). Pennsylvania State University, University Park, PA, 1980.
4. Cailliet, R: Foot and Ankle Pain, FA Davis, Philadelphia, 1968.
5. Lam, S-F, and Hodgson, ARA: A comparison of foot forms among the non-shoe and shoe-wearing Chinese population. J Bone Joint Surg 40A:1058, 1958.
6. Hardy, RH, and Clapham, JCR: Operations on hallux valgus. J Bone Joint Surg 33B:376, 1951.
7. Piggott, H: The natural history of hallux valgus in adolescence and early adult life. J Bone Joint Surg 42B:749–760, 1960.
8. Lapidus, P.W: Operative correction of the metatarsus varus primus in hallux valgus. Surg Gynecol Obstet 58:183, 1934.
9. Ellis, VH: A method of correcting metatarsus primus varus: Preliminary report. J Bone Joint Surg 33 B:415, 1951.
10. McMurray, TP: Treatment of hallux valgus and rigidus. Br Med J 2:218, 1936.
11. Inman, VT (ed): Du Vries' Surgery of the Foot, ed 3. CV Mosby, St Louis, 1973.
12. Mann, RA, and Couglin, MJ: Hallux valgus: Etiology, anatomy, treatment and surgical considerations. Clin Orthop 157:31, 1981.
13. Akin, OF: The treatment of hallux valgus: A new operative procedure and its results. Medical Sentinel 33:678, 1925.
14. Mann, RA: Surgery of the Foot. CV Mosby, St Louis, 1986, pp 89–98.
15. Selner, AJ, Ginex, SL, and Selner, MD: Tricorrectional bunionectomy for correction of high intermetatarsal angles. Am J Podiatr Med Assoc 84(8):385–389, 1994.
16. Root, ML, Orien, WP, and Weed, JH: Normal and abnormal function of the foot: Clinical biomechanics, Vol II. Clinical Biomechanics Corp., Los Angeles, 1977.

# CHAPTER 7

# The Heel

There are many reasons for a painful heel, which can be classified under three headings: (1) pain arising in tissues behind and under the heel, (2) pain arising within the bones and joints of the heel, and (3) pain arising from another source referred to the heel.

Many patients present with heel pain from numerous reasons and respond to conservative management such as rest, physical therapy, steroids, nonsteroidal anti-inflammatory medication, and orthosis without a specific diagnosis. Those who persist in their pain and disability, becoming *chronic heel pain* patients, present significant diagnostic and therapeutic problems.

## PLANTAR FASCIITIS

Pain felt under the heel and located by the patient as being "slightly ahead of the calcaneus" is frequently termed a *calcaneal heel spur*. This condition occurs in people whose recent activities have entailed prolonged standing or walking where this activity has not been previously experienced. It is noted more frequently in people who exhibit a pronated foot with a flattened longitudinal arch and who walk with a springless gait. Men are more susceptible.

Pain and local tenderness are noted beneath the anterior portion of the heel, and deep pressure reveals tenderness at the anterior medial area of the calcaneus. X-rays of the foot can be unrevealing or when prolonged may reveal a calcific spur in the anterior medial aspect of the calcaneus. A typical spur may exist in an asymptomatic person or may be absent in a symptomatic person so the diagnosis must be of the local condition and/or the presence of a spur on x-ray.

This location site of the plantar fasciitis is where the plantar fascia attaches to the anteromedial aspect of the calcaneus (Fig. 7–1). The mechanism of plan-

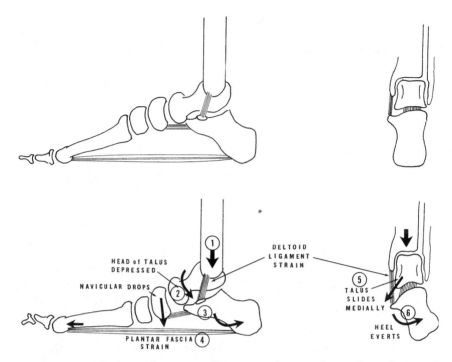

**Figure 7–1.** Mechanism and sequence of foot strain. The *upper* figures depict the normal foot with proper bone and joint alignment, adequate longitudinal arch, and a central heel. (*1*) The weight-bearing stress imparted through the tibia on the talus (*2*), which slides forward and medially (*5*) on the supporting calcaneus. The calcaneus (*3*) is depressed anteriorly, elongating the entire foot, thus placing strain on the plantar ligaments (*4*). The calcaneus everts under the downward pressure of the talus and goes into valgus (*6*).

tar fasciitis in the flat foot has been alluded to in the section on the pronated foot (Chap. 5) but merits repetition (Fig. 7–2). During gait there is repetitive traction stress on the plantar fascia and thus on the calcaneal periosteum (Fig. 7–3).

The fascia, which attaches to the periosteum of the calcaneus, is innervated by the first branch of the lateral plantar nerve. This fascia is a multilayered fibrous aponeurosis that originates from the medial calcaneal tuberosity and inserts into the plantar plates of the metatarsophalangeal joints, the flexor tendon sheaths, and the bases of the proximal phalanges of the digits. When the metatarsophalangeal joints are dorsiflexed, a windlass tightening of the plantar fascia occurs (Fig. 7–4).

Over time, numerous microtears occur in the fascia as well as some tearing away of the plantar fascial attachment to the periosteum (Fig. 7–5). Periostitis with gradual calcification results. Fatigue fractures, which can be verified by x-rays or bone scanning, may also occur.

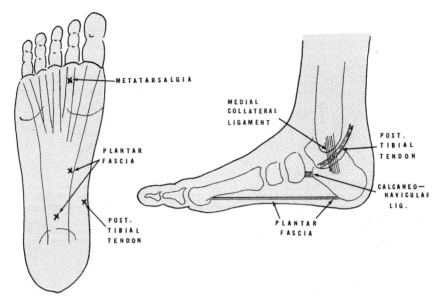

**Figure 7–2.** Tender areas in foot strain. "Trigger areas" noted in the foot undergoing strain. The initial tenderness is usually noted on the medial border of the plantar fascia and later near the heel. The deltoid ligament is not shown, but is a point of tenderness near the posterior tibial tendon, which becomes strained. The second metatarsal head is the most prevalent site of metatarsalgia.

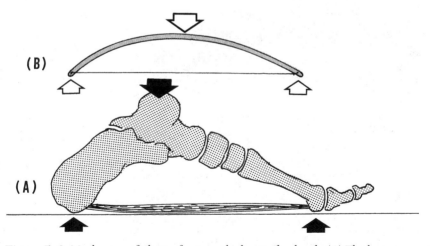

**Figure 7–3.** Mechanism of plantar fascia on the longitudinal arch. (A) The large arrow depicts the body weight on the foot. The smaller arrows depict weight bearing on the heel (*left*) and the toes (*right*). The arch is maintained by the articular structures with the plantar fascia merely reinforcing the strength of the arch. B depicts the same mechanism with regard to a stringed bow that is pressed in the direction of the white arrows, causing tension on the string (fascia).

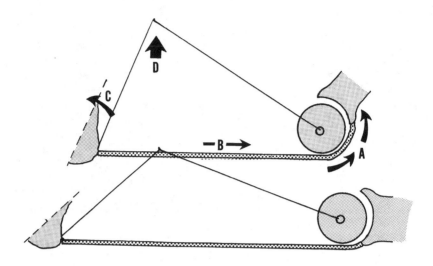

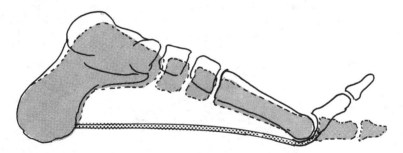

**Figure 7–4.** Effects of toes on the plantar fascia. The *lower* figure depicts the longitudinal arch, which flattens (shaded portion) on weight bearing. The *upper* figure shows (A) toe extension (curved arrow) placing tension on the plantar fascia (B) and rotation of the calcaneus (C). The longitudinal arch should increase (D) but superincumbent weight denies this elevation and instead causes strain on the fascia.

## Treatment

Local management must be instituted before resorting to surgical intervention. Because pronation is a frequent contributing factor, it must be addressed by proper orthosis. Prevention of local pressure on the calcaneal site may relieve weight-bearing pain (Fig. 7–6). However, as a traction type of injury, this type of intervention, per se, is usually ineffectual.

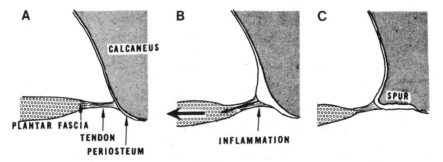

**Figure 7–5.** Mechanism of plantar fasciitis. *A* is the normal relationship of the plantar fascia with its tendon attaching to the calcaneal periosteum. *B* depicts traction (arrow) pulling the periosteum from the calcaneus. *C* shows subperiosteal invasion of inflammatory tissue, which becomes ossified, forming a spur.

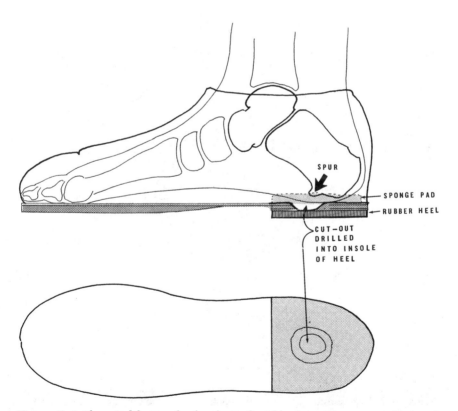

**Figure 7–6.** Shoe modification for the plantar fascial heel spur. A sponge pad inserted into the heel of the shoe decreases the pressure on the calcaneous. A cut-out can be performed into the insole of the heel of the shoe.

Injection of a local anesthetic agent and a steroid into the site of the fascial-periosteal insult is often palliative, whether it is for a local fasciitis or a nerve entrapment (Fig. 7–7).

The surgical treatment chosen is usually plantar fasciotomy and removal of the heel spur. This procedure affords inconsistent results.[1] The technique of DuVries[2] approaches the heel medially and removes the spur after approaching it between the fascial layers to allow them to remain. It was during this procedure that the nerve supply to the area, between the fascia and the abductor hallucis muscle, was revealed (Fig. 7–8).[3] It is probable that injection of an analgesic agent and steroid into the spur area affects this nerve.

The first branch of the lateral plantar nerve is a mixed motor and sensory nerve to the abductor digiti quinti muscle but also to the quadratus plantae

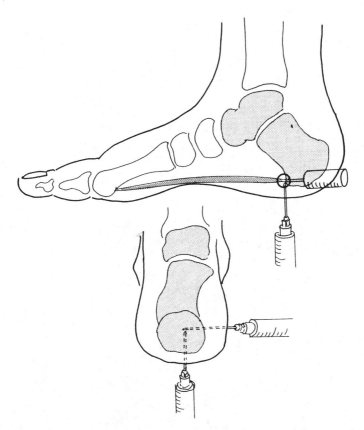

**Figure 7–7.** Injection technique in plantar fasciitis. Injection can be administered directly into the point of maximum tenderness of the plantar fascia through the heel pad. The fascia inserts into the calcaneus in this area. The site can be reached from the lateral or medial approach, but such localization is not accurate.

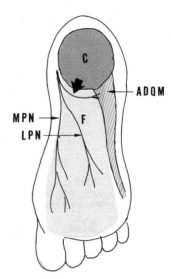

**Figure 7–8.** Nerve supply to the abductor digiti quinti muscle. The nerve supply to the abductor digiti quinti muscle (ADQM) also supplies sensation from the periosteum of the calcaneus (C) and lies under the plantar fascia (F). This nerve branch is from the lateral plantar nerve (LPN). The medial plantar nerve (MPBN) is also shown. Entrapment causing heel pain is at the large arrow.

muscle and the periosteum of the calcaneus.[4] The exact site of entrapment is between the heavy, deep fascia of the abductor hallucis muscle and the medial caudal margin of the medial head of the quadratus plantae muscle just distal to the medial calcaneal tuberosity. The nerve is decompressed by meticulous visual exposure, and postoperatively all other modalities are employed.

## PAINFUL HEEL PAD

Pain may be noted over the entire heel pad. This pad is composed of fatty tissue and elastic fibrous tissue enclosed within compartments formed by fibrous septa. Young (Fig. 7–9) tissue has an elasticity that permits the pad to act as a "shock absorber." This elasticity decreases with age or repeated trauma, causing the body weight to be borne by a less padded, or even unpadded, calcaneus. Untreated, this condition allows scar tissue to form within the compartments and the underlying periosteum to be eburnated. Compartment layers may actually rupture, allowing the fluid within the compartment to leave. Acute heel pad trauma may be the cause, as can repeated injuries.

The diagnosis is generalized heel-pad tenderness with a palpable absence or diminution of a compressible pad.

Effective treatment usually involves merely relieving pressure on the heel by inserting a sponge heel pad in the shoe or raising the heel, thus transferring the weight bearing anteriorly on stance and heel strike. Infiltration of several cubic centimeters of a local analgesic with or without steriods may relieve the symptoms. The condition happily is usually self-limited.

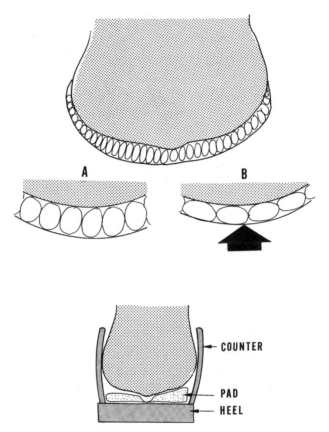

**Figure 7–9.** Heel pad. The heel pad encloses the entire posterior-inferior aspect of the calcaneus and is formed of numerous "cells" of contained fluid. These pads (A) expand with no weight bearing and compress (B) with weight bearing. With injury, these cells can rupture, thus losing their contour. Treatment is to replace the pad as indicated in the *lower* figure.

## DUPUYTREN'S CONTRACTURE

Dupuytren's contracture similiar to that found in the hand may occur within the plantar fascia (see Fig. 7–1). This syndrome presents lobulated, firm nodules within the plantar fascia. These "tumors" are fibrous, and biopsy reveals cellular components of proliferating fibroblasts. They are adherent to the skin, causing puckering of the skin. They grow slowly and cause mechanical concern. The nodules develop within the fatty tissue superficial to the plantar aponeurosis with fibrous bands extending centrifugally from the nodules. Progression may cease at any time with no apparent reason found. The nodules may be confused with fibrosarcoma and must be carefully differentiated by a competent pathologist.

Heredity is a factor in Dupuytren's contracture[5,6] with repeated trauma considered less probable. This condition becomes more prominent in the fourth decade of life and is more prevalent in alcoholic, epileptic, and diabetic patients. It is more prevalent in patients with increased sympathetic tone and predisposition to reflex sympathetic dystrophy.

## ACHILLES PERITENDINITIS

The structure of the tendon has been well documented.[7] It is composed of parallel bands of collagen fibers (Figs. 7–10 through 7–12) that curl and uncurl as they are subjected to traction forces. On release of these forces, if physiologic, they recoil to their original length.[8–10] Repeated elongation of tension causes a collagen fiber to "creep," which implies a slight yet physiologic elongation.

When injured, connective tissue is repaired by accumulation of inflammatory cells with stimulation of microphages and formation of fibroblasts that synthesize collagen. These fibroblasts also form *scar*. Fibroblasts are usually the sole cellular component of adult tendons, with collagen the major component of the extracellular matrix.

Achilles tendinitis is probably more correctly termed *peritendinitis*. Inflammation of the tendon occurs near the insertion of the tendon some 4 to 8 cm above the calcaneus. The condition is not tenosynovitis since the Achilles tendon has no synovial tendon sheath. Inflammation occurs within the loose connective tissue known as *paratenon*.

Trauma or stress is the usual cause. Clinically the tendon is tender on being squeezed between the examiner's fingers. There may be some thickening, but usually none is noted. Stretching the tendon causes pain.

Treatment consists of resting the part and preventing elongation of the tendon. This means eliminating gastrocnemius-soleus muscle activities. Casting the foot and ankle in a below-the-knee cast for 4 weeks usually allows healing. Casting is then followed by gentle, progressive elongation and gradual gastrocnemius-soleus exercises. Injecting an analgesic and soluble steroid into the ten-

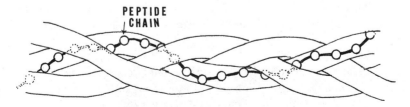

**Figure 7–10.** Tropocollagen trihelix fiber.

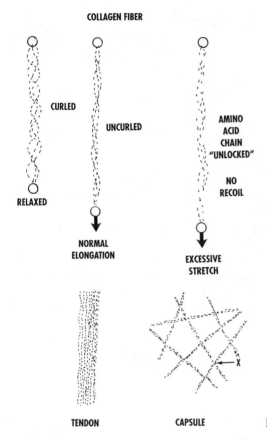

**Figure 7–11.** Collagen fibers.

don has its advocates. The tendon remains prone to further damage and even rupture, so doing strengthening exercises and minimizing trauma are pertinent.

## RUPTURE OF ACHILLES TENDON

After a stressful event, acute posterior calf pain along with having heard a "snap" indicates a potential tear of the Achilles tendon. The mechanism of tearing is from acute excessive contraction of the gastrocnemius-soleus muscle group or a direct external blow to the contracted gastrocnemius-soleus tendon complex.

Ecchymosis is usually noted, and the tear may be palpable (Fig. 7–13). A test has been postulated to determine the completeness of the tear. This is termed the *Simmond's test*. With the patient prone and both feet protruding over the edge of the table, the calf muscles are squeezed. In the normal foot, the ankle plantar flexes, whereas in the partially torn side, there is no, or at least

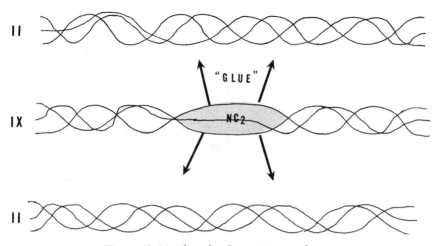

**Figure 7–12.** The role of type IX in cartilage.

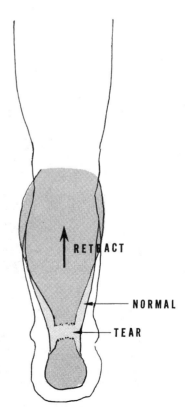

**Figure 7–13.** Torn Achilles tendon. Most Achilles tendon tears are complete and occur approximately 2 inches above the calcaneal insert. The calf muscle retracts toward the popliteal space and a "gap" often can be felt at the site of the tear. Patient cannot rise on tiptoes.

diminished, plantar flexion. In the erect position, the patient cannot arise on the toes of the affected leg.

Rupture of the Achilles tendon was first described by Ambrose Paré in 1575 and again in 1768 by Hunter, who sustained a rupture while dancing. Hunter treated himself with strapping and raised heel with apparent good results,[11] a form of treatment still advocated.

If intervention is indicated, it must be done early because substantial granulation in the gap, which prevents approximation of the torn ends, occurs within a week.[12] Without surgical repair, rerupture occurs in approximately 10% to 29% of cases, whereas after surgical repair, only 2% recur.[13] Buck[14] sectioned a rat's Achilles tendon and allowed it to retract without suture. A fibrin coagulum was randomly laid down in the defect between the torn ends (Fig. 7–14).

Within 4 days, fibroblasts began to grow into the coagulum from the periphery. Gradually, the collagen fibers became oriented in a parallel manner along a longitudinal direction. Within 2 weeks the entire length of the tendon up to the muscular insertion was invaded by fibroblasts. It is apparent that healing occurs in human adults within 24 months, but the tendon may not be of sufficient normal length or strength.

The overlying skin may tether, causing an inflexible scar that prejudices healing, skin necrosis, and even infection. Skin expansion by a soft-tissue

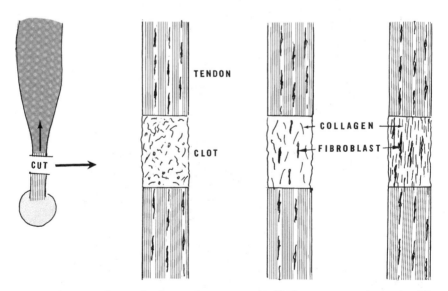

**Figure 7–14.** Tendon cut healing without suture. (*Left*) The cut area in the tendon fills with a fibrin clot. Fibroblasts enter the clot and initiate formation of collagen fibers. (*Middle*) At first, these are random in direction, but gradually they become longitudinally aligned (*right*), as are normal collagen fibers. (Modified from Buck, RC: Regeneration of tendon. J Pathol Bacteriol 16:1–18, 1953.)

expander assists in preventing this sequela.[15] Postoperative reduction of muscle power may be brought about by disuse atrophy or a failure to restore the original tendon length. The former can be restored by exercise, but the latter has an unfavorable prognosis.[16]

## GASTROCNEMIUS MUSCLE TEAR

The Achillles tendon rupture usually occurs at the junction of the gastrocnemius-soleus tendon complex, whereas a tear of the gastrocnemius muscle usually occurs in the medial head of the muscle (Fig. 7–15). Most occur usually in the 30 to 50 years age group.

In a torn tendon, the Thompson test is positive, which means that the ankle plantar does not plantar flex from squeezing the calf. In a gastrocnemius muscle tear, there is no palpable defect in the muscle-tendon complex and the Thompson test is negative; that is, the foot and ankle plantar flex from calf squeeze.

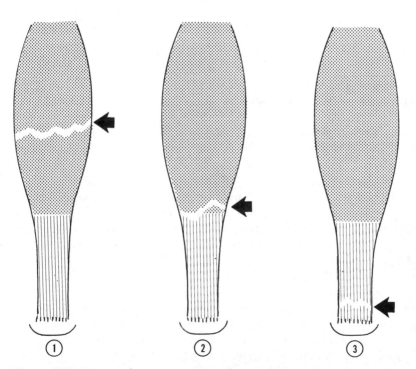

**Figure 7–15.** Tears in the gastrocnemius-soleus tendon complex. (*1*) A muscle tear in the medial gastrocnemius-soleus muscle; (*2*) a tear where the gastrocnemius-soleus muscle attaches to the Achilles tendon; and (*3*) a tear within the Achilles tendon proper.

Treatment involves avoiding running, jumping, and doing toe lifts and push-off activities for 4 to 6 weeks. Local ice massage and gradual, gentle stretching as tolerated are recommended. The condition is self-limited.[17]

## POSTERIOR CALCANEAL BURSITIS

Pain and tenderness of the posterior aspect of the heel and under the skin, especially occurring in women who wear high heels and narrow-counter shoes, are caused by a bursal inflammation that occurs between the tendon and the skin. The inflamed bursa is usually visible with the skin overlying it reddened and the bursa swollen and palpable. If allowed to become chronic, the skin thickens, as does the wall of the bursa. All become adherent.

Treatment is the removal of the inflaming shoe. The posterior aspect of the shoe counter can be cut out, or a moleskin patch can be placed over the bursa between the inner wall of the shoe counter. Local modalities to the inflamed bursa are indicated, as are antibiotics. Aspiration under sterile conditions often is needed to drain the bursa. The drainage may be followed by insertion of a soluble steroid.

## CALCANEAL APOPHYSITIS

Also known as *Sever's disease*, calcaneal apophysitis is a painful condition of children before their epiphyses close. It occurs most often in active adolescent males between the age of 8 and 13 years. It occurs from excessive trauma caused by stress to the Achilles tendon in jumping activities. It has been classified under the general osteochondroses syndromes, which include Calvé-Legg-Perthes disease of the hip and Osgood-Schlatter disease of the tibial tuberosity. The latter is considered a traction injury of an unfused epiphysis.

The diagnosis is suggested when a teenager complains of pain and tenderness at the back of the heel below the attachment of the Achilles tendon. Walking may be completely pain free, and the condition, usually unilateral, may be bilateral. The localized pain is tender on touch and pressure. There may be swelling and redness over the area, and pain is aggravated by standing and arising on tiptoes or by jumping.

In the early phase, x-rays are nondiagnostic because the usual fragmented apophysis is similiar to the normal side. Difference in fragmentation may be suggestive. Bone scanning will ultimately reveal inflammation at the site. MRI could be diagnostic, but that expensive study is rarely indicated.

Treatment is symptomatic since the condition is usually self-limited and, unless extreme, leaves no residual functional defect. Curtailing activities that cause Achilles stretch are indicated, even though this is difficult to enforce in active males of that age. A shoe heel lift of up to $1/4$ inch places the foot in equinus and lessens the Achilles strain. Crutches are valuable if the condition is unilateral and severe. In severe conditions, a walking plaster cast that extends above the knee and places the foot in slight equinus is indicated. The parents can be reassured that the condition is not of severe potential disability, once the inflammation has subsided.

## SUBTALAR ARTHRITIS

Pain felt "within the heel" may be referred from an arthritic subtalar joint. This arthritic condition may result from trauma such as occurs in a calcaneal fracture. The diagnosis of *subtalar arthritis* is made by pain elicited from passive motion of the subtalar joint, which has been previously described (see Chap. 2). Crepitation as well as pain may be elicited, and there may be tenderness from deep pressure into the tarsal tunnel opening directly in front of the lateral malleolus with the foot inverted. X-rays reveal damage to the talocalcaneal joint. Weight bearing is painful, and local rest affords relief.

Treatment consists of local rest and anti-inflammation medication.

Little attention has been given to subtalar instability after a severe ankle ligamentous sprain. Ligamentous instability does occur in this joint (see Fig. 7–17). The motion of this joint can be tested by passively dorsiflexing the foot, which immobilizes the talus within the mortise. Then manual passive motion of the calcaneus tests the stability of the talocalcaneal joint.

Treatment consists of local rest and anti-inflammation modalities. Casting affords relief if the condition is severe. Local injection of a steroid and analgesic into the tarsal tunnel also affords temporary relief (Figs. 7–16 and 7–17). A molded orthosis is effective. Surgical fusion of the talocalcaneal joint is offered if all else fails and the disability is significant.

## JOGGER'S FOOT PAIN

Today, with both athletes and nonathletes performing numerous, daily, stressful physical activities, the *jogger's foot* is a frequent complaint (Fig. 7–18). In addition to impact injuries to the heel pad and the metatarsal heads, the fit of athletic shoes may also be traumatic, causing bunion inflammation.

The lower leg has four muscle compartments: the anterior, lateral, superficial posterior, and deep posterior. The *anterior* contains the tibialis anterior, extensor digitorum longus, extensor hallucis longus, and peroneus tertius muscles. The *lateral compartment* contains the peroneus longus and brevis muscles. The *superficial posterior compartment* contains the gastrocnemius-soleus muscle complex, and the *deep posterior compartment* includes the posterior tibialis, flexor hallucis longus, and flexor digitorum longus muscles.

A *compartment syndrome* is an acute increase in tissue pressure within an enclosed anatomic space in which the enclosed muscles are bounded by *semirigid* fascia. Normal intracompartmental pressure with the muscles at rest is

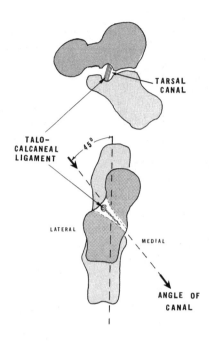

**Figure 7–16.** Talocalcaneal joint. The talus and calcaneus are joined by three facets: anterior, middle, and posterior. The tarsal tunnel in its oblique course (sulcus) contains the talocalcaneal ligaments.

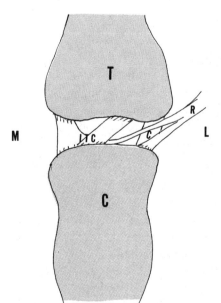

**Figure 7–17.** Ligamentous complex of the talocalcaneal joint. The talus (T) and calcaneus (C) form the talocalcaneal joint. It is connected by a capsule (not shown) and the interosseous talocalcaneal ligament (ITC), cervical (c) ligament, and retinaculum (R).

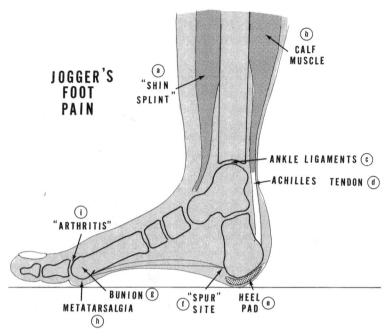

**Figure 7–18.** Jogger's foot pain. The foot, ankle, and lower leg pains sustained by jogger's are shown: (a) "Shin splints": myositis of anterior tibialis muscle; (b) calf pain; (c) talotibial ligamentous strain; (d) Achilles tendon strain; (e) inflamed heel pad; (f) plantar fascia strain, causing "spur"-type pain; (g) bunion pain, if a hallux valgus exists; (h) metatarsalgia; and (i) arthralgia of the big toe metatarsophalangeal joint.

0 to 10 mm Hg. Increased local pressure occludes venous return, which gradually leads to a decrease in the arteriovenous gradient, and then to a decrease in arterial flow. A pressure of 30 mm Hg indicates impending syndrome, and a pressure of 30 to 40 mm Hg is ominous and needs careful monitoring and treatment.

The initial symptoms of compartment syndrome are pain on active and passive stretching of the muscles within the compartment. There is local tenderness. Later symptoms are hypesthesia from the compressed nerves within the compartment and weakness of the enclosed muscles.

In general, treatment of a compression syndrome consists of removal of circular dressing, elevation of the limb, and surgical decompression if pressure persists. If untreated, irreversible necrosis of the muscles is the end result.

In athletic activities, the muscular component of the lower leg poses problems such as "shin splints" and painful gastrocnemius-soleus muscle strain. The *shin splint* is an inflammatory condition of the muscles within the anterior compartment (Fig. 7–19).[18–20] Shin splints often occur early in the season in an untrained individual, using poorly fitted, inappropriate shoes, running on hard surfaces, and engaging in excessive initial activity.

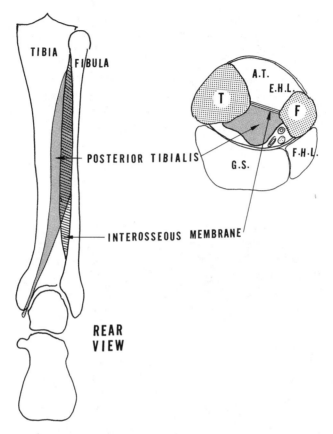

**Figure 7–19.** The anterior compartment. The lower leg is divided into several compartments containing muscle groups within semiflexible fascial sheaths, of which the interosseous membrane between the tibia (T) and the fibula (F) is predominant. The anterior compartment contains the anterior tibialis muscle (AT) and the extensor hallucis longus (EHL). The posterior compartment is less confined and contains the gastrocnemius-soleus muscle (GS) and the flexor hallucis longus (FHL). Other muscles are found in the lower leg (see accompanying text).

Treatment initially includes rest with icing and anti-inflammatory medication. When severe and prolonged, anterior fasciotomy may be necessary to decompress the compartment.

*Medial tibial stress syndrome* (MTSS) is an inflammatory condition involving the periosteum of the deep posterior compartment. This differs from shin splints as to its tissue site. Pain usually starts after exercise, and there is tenderness over the posterior medial edge of the distal third of the tibia. Radiographs are usually nondiagnostic. Foot pronation predisposes one to this condition. Treatment includes initially rest and local modalities such as ice and then heat.

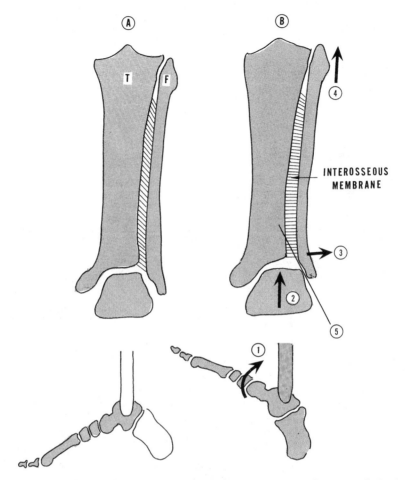

**Figure 7–20.** Effect of foot dorsiflexion on the interosseous membrane. With the foot in neutral position (*A*), the membrane fibers are angled. As the foot (*B*) dorsiflexes (1) and places the anterior border of the talus (2) between the malleoli, the lateral malleolus (3) moves laterally and the fibula ascends (4), causing the membrane fibers to become elongated and horizontal. Heel cord stretching exercise thus elongates this membrane as well as elongates the gastrocnemius-soleus muscle tendon complex.

Exercises to strengthen and increase the flexibility of the deep posterior compartment muscles are encouraged to prevent recurrence. Heel-cord stretching also stretched the interosseous membrane (Fig. 7–20), which is needed. Then foot pronation must be addressed.

*Chronic exertional compartment syndrome* has been designated as a painful syndrome that occurs "only during" exercise with symptoms that subside on cessation of the exercise. Some numbness of the foot and ankle may persist. This must be monitored carefully because it indicates an elevation of intra-compartmental pressure with gradual diminution on cessation of exercise. In 50% to 60% of patients, these compartment syndromes are bilateral.

## FRACTURES OF THE OS CALCIS

It has been generally accepted that the results of fractures of the calcaneus are severe, with recovery slow and incomplete.[21] There is disagreement as to classification of the types of fracture with a practical classification indicating whether there is fracture *without* involvement of the subtalar joint or fracture *with* joint involvement. This classification obviously involves proper interpretation of the x-rays.

Nonoperative treatment results in an unsatisfactory outcome in 30% to 50% of patients, but operated-on patients report unsatisfactory results in 25% to 40%, a small encouragement.

A standard protocol for evaluating results has been proposed.[22] These include pain level, work and daily living activity level, sports and recreational activity level, and walking distances with aids or without, on smooth or uneven surfaces. These are subjective. Objective criteria include ankle range of motion, subtalar range of motion, limp, height of heel, arch angle, tendoachilles fulcrum length, and length of the calcaneus. These criteria do not indicate radiologic end results.

Whether choosing operative or nonoperative management, the major goal for ensuring a good result is to achieve early range of motion. Non-weight-bearing for 8 to 12 weeks prevents collapse of the surgically reduced and fixed bones and joint, yet allows dystrophic changes to occur, which may be pain producing. Traction of the calcaneus with insertion of a graft to ensure proper length has been proposed.[23] The techniques of surgical procedure are beyond the scope of this text.[24]

## REFERENCES

1. Baxter, DE, Pfeffer, GB, and Thigpen, M: Chronic heel pain: Management of foot problems. Orthop Clin North Am 20(4):563–569, 1989.
2. DuVries, HL: Heel spur (calcaneal spur). Arch Surg 74:536–542, 1957.
3. Graham, CE: Painful heel syndrome: Rationale of diagnosis and treatment. Foot Ankle 2(5):261–267, 1983.
4. Rondhuis, JJ, and Huson, A: The first branch of the lateral plantar nerve and heel pain. Acta Morphol Neerl Scand 24:269–280, 1986.
5. Larsen, RD, and Posch, JL: Dupuytren's contracture with special reference to pathology. J Bone Joint Surg 40A:773, 1958.
6. Sigler, JW: Dupuytren's contracture, Chap. 81. In Hollander, SE, and McCarty, DFJ (eds): Arthritis and Allied Conditions, ed. 8. Lea & Febiger, Philadelphia, 1972, pp 1503–1510.

7. Cailliet, R: Soft tissue concepts, Chap. 1. In Soft Tissue Pain and Disability, ed 3. FA Davis, Philadelphia, 1996.

8. Rigby, BJ, Hirai, N, and Spikes, JD: The mechanical behavior of rat tail tendon. J Gen Physiol 43:265–283, 1959.

9. Van Brocklin, JD, and Ellis, DG: A study of the mechanical behavior of toe extensor tendons under applied stress. Arch Phys Med Rehabil 46:369–370, 1965.

10. Noyes, FR, et al: Biomechanics of ligament failure. II. An analysis of immobilization, exercise, and reconditioning effects in primates. J Bone Joint Surg (Am) 56:1406–1417, 1974.

11. Kobler, J: The Reluctant Surgeon: A Biography of John Hunter. Doubleday, New York, 1906, pp. 249–250.

12. Arner, O, and Lindholm, A: Subcutaneous rupture of the Achilles tendon: A study of 92 cases. Acta Chir Scand Suppl 239:1–51, 1959.

13. Carden, DG, et al: Rupture of calcaneal tendon: The early and late management. J Bone Joint Surg (Br) 69B:416–420, 1987.

14. Buck, RC: Regeneration of tendon. J Pathol Bacteriol 66:1–18, 1953.

15. Mohammed, A, Rahamatalla, A, and Wynne-Jones, CH: Tissue expansion in late repair of tendo Achilles rupture. J Bone Joint Surg 77B(1): 64–66, 1995.

16. Kakiuchi M: A combined open and percutaneous technique for repair of tendo Achilles. J Bone Joint Surg 77B(1):60–63, 1995.

17. Shields, CL, Redix, L, and Brewster, CE: Acute tears of the medial head of the gastrocnemius. Foot Ankle 5:186, 1985.

18. Brown, DE: Lower leg syndromes. In Mellion, MB (ed): Sports Medicine Secrets. Hanley & Belfus, Philadelphia, 1994, pp 304–307.

19. Pedowitz, RA, et al: Modified criteria for the objective diagnosis of chronic compartment syndrome of the leg. Am J Sports Med 18:35, 1990.

20. Styf, JR, and Korner, LM: Chronic anterior compartment syndrome of the leg: Results of treatment by fasciotomy. J Bone Joint Surg 68A:1338, 1986.

21. Essex-Lopresti, P: The mechanism, reduction technique, and results in fractures of the os calcis. Clin Orthop Rel Res 290:3–16, 1993.

22. Paley, D, and Hall, H: Calcaneal fracture controversies: Can we put Humpty Dumpty together again? Orthop Clin North Am 20(4):665–677, 1989.

23. Carr, J, Hansen, S, and Benirschke, S: Subtalar distraction bone block fusion for late complicatons of os calcis fractures. Foot Ankle 9:81, 1988.

24. Hammesfahr, JFR: Surgical treatment of calcaneal fractures. Orthop Clin North Am 20(4):679–689, 1989.

# CHAPTER 8

# Injuries to the Ankle

## ANKLE JOINT

The ankle joint depends on support from the medial and lateral collateral ligaments (Figs. 8–1 to 8–3). The ankle joint is stable because of the mechanical configuration of the joint as well (see Figs. 1–2 through 1–5) as the ligamentous support. The tibiofibular ligament is also active during ankle motion (Fig. 8–4). When the foot dorsiflexes and plantar flexes at the ankle, the talus spreads the tibia and fibula to the extent allowed by the tibiofibular ligament.

Stability is afforded to the ankle joint by the above-mentioned ligaments: varus is limited by the lateral collateral ligament and valgus by the medial (Fig. 8–5).

Anterior displacement (shear) of the leg on the foot is also limited by the tendons and ligaments that cross the foot (see Fig. 1–10). The talus has no muscles attached to it. It fits snugly into the mortise formed by the malleoli of the tibia and the fibula. In the dorsiflexion position, the broader anterior portion of the talus is forced between the two malleoli, spreading the fibula and tibia as far as the interosseous ligament of the lower leg will permit (see Fig. 8–4). In dorsiflexion, there is no significant motion of the talus within the mortise in either varus or valgus of the foot.

In plantar flexion, the talus presents its narrowest portion between the two malleoli and thus permits lateral motion of the foot in either varus or valgus motion. Some motion of the talus is permitted with the foot in a neutral position. Other than during extreme dorsiflexion, the ligaments of the ankle are subjected to stress when varus or valgus is imposed on the foot-ankle complex.

The medial collateral ligaments have an eccentric axis of rotation (see Fig. 8–3) so that all fibers are taut in the neutral position; however, the pos-

202

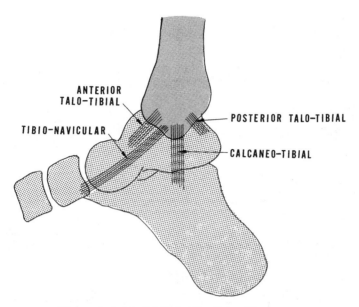

**Figure 8–1.** Medial (deltoid) collateral ligaments.

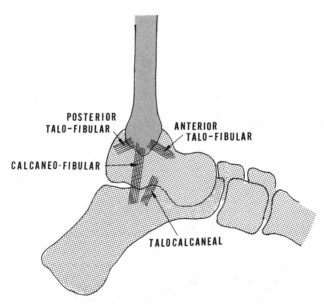

**Figure 8–2.** Lateral collateral ligaments.

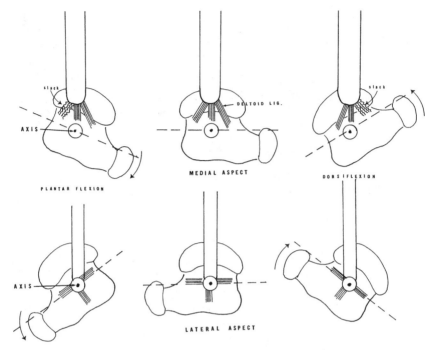

**Figure 8–3.** Relationship of medial and lateral collateral ligaments to axis of rotation of ankle. In the medial aspect of the ankle, the axis of rotation is eccentric to the medial collateral ligaments and thus they vary in length with ankle motion as shown. Because the axis of rotation is central on the lateral side, the length of the ligaments does not vary.

terior fibers are relaxed in plantar flexion and the anterior fibers in dorsiflexion. The lateral collateral ligaments have a central axis of rotation; thus all fibers remain taut in all ranges of plantar flexion and dorsiflexion.

The ligaments run from the malleoli to the talus, calcaneus, and navicular. They are well supplied by sensory nerves, which subserve proprioception and mediate pain when the flexibility of ligaments is exceeded or damaged.

## Ankle Ligamentous Injuries

Ankle ligamentous injury occurs when the leg moves beyond the confines of the ligamentous support within the mortise. As the reflex mechanism of tendinous innervation with resultant instantaneous musculoskeletal contraction is not possible, instability of the ankle occurs.

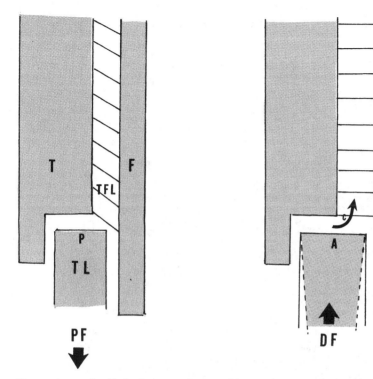

**Figure 8–4.** Tibiofibular ligament during ankle motion. In the *left* figure, with the ankle plantar flexed (PF), the posterior, narrower portion of the talus (P) is between the tibia (T) and the fibula (F), allowing the tibiofibular ligament (TFL) to remain oblique. During ankle dorsiflexion (DF) in *right* figure, the fibula ascends (a) and moves laterally (b), causing the tibiofibular ligamentous fibers to become horizontal to their full elongation.

## Clinical Evaluation

Injury to the lateral ankle ligaments in an ankle sprain is the most common sports-incurred injury. Sixteen percent of sports injuries recorded in an Oslo hospital emergency room were ankle sprains.[1] Another report[2] noted that 45% of basketball injuries were sustained by the ankle.

There are three principal lateral ankle ligaments—the anterior talofibular, calcaneofibular, and posterior talofibular—that form the lateral collateral ligaments of the ankle that sustain athletic injury. The anterofibular ligament (ATFL) is the weakest and the most often injured. The calcaneofibular ligament (CFL) is the next weakest but is 2½ times stronger than the ATFL. The posterior talofibular ligament (PTFL) has twice the strength of the ATFL.[3]

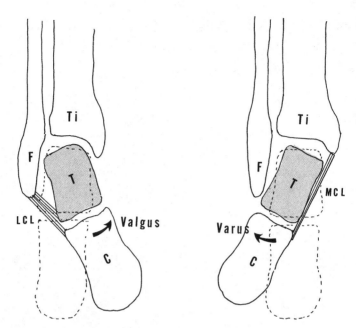

**Figure 8–5.** Medial-lateral displacement of the ankle. *Left*, with the foot going into valgus, the talus (T) and the calcaneus (C) displace in a medial direction related to the tibia (Ti) and the fibula (F). This places stress on the lateral collateral ligaments (LCL). *Right*, when the foot moves into varus, the opposite action of the talus and calcaneus occurs, placing stress on the medial collateral ligaments (MCL).

Because the ATFL is involved in plantar flexion and internal rotation, it is the most often injured. In plantar flexion, its fibers are oriented at 75° to the floor; in ballet dancers who achieve greater plantar flexion, the ATFL may be totally vertical to the floor (Fig. 8–6). At this degree of plantar flexion, the talus is the most flexible position within the ankle mortise. The ATFL has been shown to provide stability against talar tilt.[4]

The ATFL and PTFL both blend with the ankle capsule. The CFL does not. Injury of the first two therefore also incurs a capsular reaction. Because of its relationship with the blunt end of the fibula (see Fig. 8–6), the ATFL usually tears in its midsection (Fig. 8–7).

The PTFL, which is the strongest ligament on the lateral aspect of the ankle, is oriented horizontally and thus is the least often injured. The CFL ligament is a rounded ligament that stabilizes the talus on the calcaneus in severe ankle varus injuries.

In normal gait with normal ankles, there is normal ligamentous stress during all phases of gait. With ligamentous injury, there is excessive internal rotation during gait.

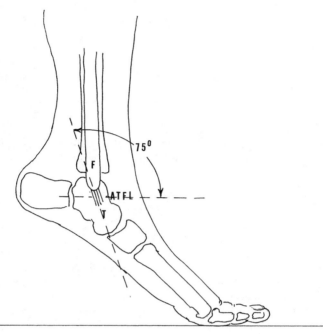

**Figure 8–6.** Direction of the anteriotalar-fibular ligament in plantar flexion. In dancers who elevate with extreme plantar flexion, the ankle ligaments are susceptible to injury when the anterior talo-fibular ligament (ATFL) is almost verticle (75°—dashed line) to the floor. F is the fibular malleolus, and T the talus.

## Mechanism of Injury

At foot (toe) strike, the foot is plantar flexed and supinated (see Chap. 2), causing the talus to be movable within the mortise, placing stress on the ligaments. If there is rotational or lateral stress from the activity, the lateral ligaments are overwhelmed and sustain injury of varying grades.[5]

Commonly the exact specifics of the injury are not recalled because they have occurred during a rapid athletic activity. In retrospect, the weight-bearing foot that sustains the injury undergoes inversion stress as the other leg activates the stress. Frequently, the foot-ankle "gives way" and is immediately followed by pain; swelling at the lateral malleolus and ecchymosis is noted.

The examination reveals the following:

1. Tenderness over the lateral ankle ligaments immediately below the lateral malleolus.
2. Swelling and ecchymosis.

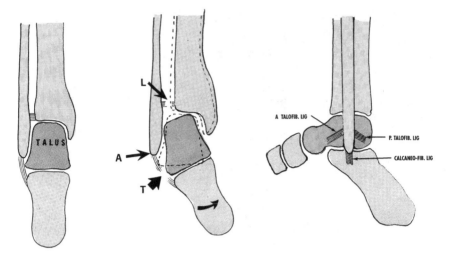

**Figure 8–7.** Lateral collateral ligament tear. The *left* figure shows the normal ankle from an anterior view and the *right* figure from a lateral view. The *middle* figure shows a severe inversion injury of the talus and calcaneus (curved arrow), which causes a talar tilt, tearing the lateral collateral ligament (T), possible avulsion (A) of the fibular malleolus, and possible tear of the interosseous ligament (L).

3. Pain is increased by inversion of the foot-ankle, and there is significantly greater motion than that noted in the opposite foot-ankle (Fig. 8–8).
4. The anterior drawer test must be performed to determine sagittal stability (Fig. 8–9).
5. The stability of the talocalcaneal ligament must be tested (see Fig. 5–17).
6. Rotational instability may also be tested. This is performed by having the patient lie prone. The 90° flexed knee permits testing rotation of the foot-ankle, and then comparing the range after testing the opposite foot-ankle.

In common ankle sprains, complete tears occur in 75%, with two-thirds occurring at the ATFL[4] in the midsection. Two-thirds were isolated ATFL injuries, and 20% had a concomitant CFL tear. Only 14% had an avulsion injury. The amount of instability also correlated with the degree of capsular tear.

Radiologic studies are implemented to rule out fracture and/or avulsion. Stress films have been advocated as has arthrography, but these have been questioned as to their accuracy.[6]

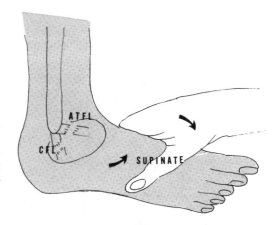

**Figure 8–8.** Inversion stress test of ankle. To test the integrity of the lateral collateral ligaments, the inversion test shown supinates the foot (curved arrows), causing excessive motion as compared with normal. There is tenderness over the lateral malleolus where the anterior talofibular ligament (ATFL) and the calcaneofibular ligament (CFL) are located.

## Treatment

Despite their frequency, the treatment of ankle sprains remains controversial, especially the treatment of grade III (severe) ligamentous injuries.[3]

The severity of an ankle sprain is so frequently unrecognized that the statement of Watson-Jones[8] must be heeded: "It is worse to sprain an ankle than to break it." The implication is that sprains are often neglected and inadequately treated.

Treatment of the acute, grades I and II sprains has been essentially as follows[9]:

1. Local ice, elevation, compression dressing, and crutches for at least the first 24 hours (Fig. 8–10).
2. Early active motion within the compression stocking of dorsiflexion and plantar flexion exercises.
3. Gradually, toe raises and eversion-inversion exercises against increasing resistance.
4. Casting and wrapping with an elastic bandage has its advocates, but "how long" remains controversial.

With grade II injuries, controversy surrounds the use of early surgical intervention, which has been advocated, especially for young, active athletes.[10]

---

°Classification of ankle ligamentous injuries:

*Grade I*: Minor ligamentous injury with maintenance of functional integrity. There is minimal functional loss, little swelling and tenderness, and mild pain on stress.

*Grade II*: Moderate sprain. Nearly complete ligamentous disruption is present. There is moderate functional loss with difficulty toe walking, diffuse swelling, and tenderness.

*Grade III*: Complete ligamentous rupture with marked functional disability, marked tenderness, swelling, and pain.[7]

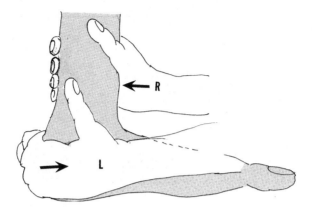

**Figure 8–9.** Sagittal stress test of ankle: "Drawer sign." Holding the lower leg (R, right hand), the other hand (L) pulls the entire foot anteriorly. Excessive motion is a positive "drawer sign," indicating a tear of the anterior talofibular ligament when compared to the other normal side.

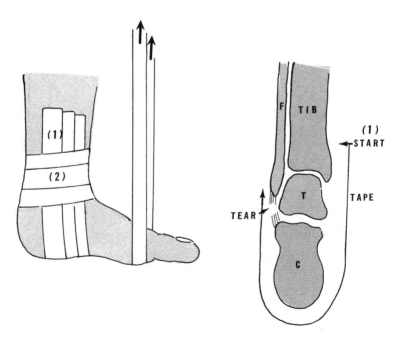

**Figure 8–10.** Taping a sprained ankle. The strap around the forefoot (two vertical arrows) dorsiflexes the foot but also inverts or everts the foot as needed before taping. Vertical tapes (1) invert or evert the ankle as indicated by the curved arrow (tape). Horizontal tapes (2) minimize rotation as well as firming the vertical taping.

Residual pain and instability have been found in 20% to 40% of those treated conservatively, whereas 90% of patients treated surgically have good results. Patients with avulsion fractures and associated fractures usually benefit from surgical intervention.

## Ligament Healing

Because the goal of all therapeutic approaches is to regain ligament ankle stability, the healing time of the ligaments must be ascertained. Most ligament healing times have been determined for cruciate knee ligaments, with few relating to the ankle. However, ligaments, per se, have been studied. Clayton and colleagues[11] determined that sutured and unsutured ligaments heal to be stronger than normal osseous ligaments at their juncture, but these were not tested by stress.

Mechanical behavioral studies of ligaments have involved elongating tendons until they ruptured while measuring length and tension during stretch. This has led to a *stress-strain curve*.[12] *Recovery* occurs after stress is removed, *before* rupture. *Creep* is the slow elongation in response to constant or repeated stress. After tearing, changes in recovery have been experimentally documented.[12,13]

Macrophages occur at the edge of the tear, followed by newborn fibroblasts. These fibroblasts replicate around capillary buds and gradually mature. Microfibroblasts appear 24 to 48 hours after leukocytes appear. By 72 hours, collagen fibers appear.

The clot that appears in the space created by the tear is the site of cellular infiltration. Then collagen synthesis occurs; the collagen gradually reorganizes into parallel bands, which are thickened by the formation of fibrous scar. Tension applied during these stages of organization aligns the strands into parallel bands, hence the value of elongation exercises during healing.

## Ankle Instability

After what is considered appropriate ligament healing, a degree of instability may remain in approximately 20% to 40% of patients. It is thought that this instability occurs because of disruption of the normal glide of the talus during gait, increased subtalar motion, and increased rotation of the tibia on the talus. These changes ultimately result in degenerative changes in the articulations between the talus and the tibia.[14]

Instability undoubtedly occurs because of loss of proprioception.[15] Proprioception has been studied in the knee cruciate ligaments and in the medial collateral ligaments,[16-19] but similiar studies have not been done on the ankle.

Treatment of late ankle instability is less controversial than is the treatment of the acute injury. Reconstructive procedures have given good results in 90%

of cases,[20] whether the repair is done early or not.[21] The types of surgery are well documented[3] but are beyond the scope of this text.

## Rehabilitation

A three-phase program has been advocated for rehabilitation[9]: (1) limitation of the injury, (2) restoration of range of motion, and (3) regaining agility, balance, and endurance. For limitation of injury, a brace (Fig. 8–11) has proved effective. A brace can be used while other measures are being implemented.

For restoration of balance, which implies needing to improve proprioception, the *tilt board* has been effective (Figs. 8–12 through 8–14). The person stands with feet parallel to the underlying board at varying distances or straddles the board at varying degrees of angulation to the underboard.

If found limited, the heel cord must be stretched (see Fig. 5–43). The peroneal muscle must also be strengthened, as must the gastrocnemius-soleus

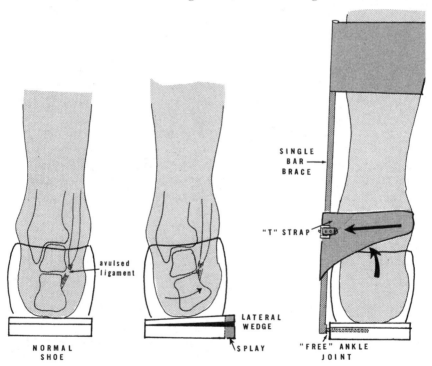

**Figure 8–11.** Bracing in conservative management of chronic dislocation of the ankle. When rehabilitation treatment for an unstable ankle is begun, the instability can be treated with a short leg brace: a single bar fastened to the shoe with a "free" ankle joint. A T strap stabilizes the ankle, and a lateral heel wedge positions the foot in varus to relieve the strain upon the lateral collateral ligaments.

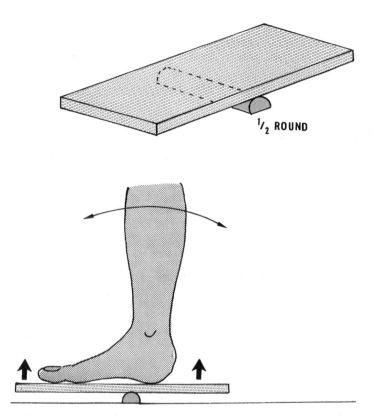

**1/₂ ROUND**

**Figure 8–12.** Tilt board. A board with a centrally placed vertical board of varying height can restore proprioception for the chronically impaired ankle. Two-leg stance or one-leg stance is determined by the needs of the patient and the severity of the residual injury.

muscle. The former is done with the foot side lying, raising a weight attached to the shoe. The latter is done by rising up on the toes with increasing frequency.

For athletes, weekend or professional, walking in a "bounce gait" at increasing speeds and duration is initiated. Jumping and then hopping is begun with increasing height, frequency, and duration. Running, at first in a straight direction and then in figure 8, may be considered for the dedicated athlete.

## SUBTALAR JOINT

Chronic lateral ligament instability has been considered at length in the medical literature, but instability of the subtalar joint as a sequela of lateral ligament instability has been considered to a lesser degree. This condition, termed *talar tilt* and *subtalar tilt*, is now found more frequently.

A tibial calcaneal angle of ±38° has been considered normal (Fig. 8–15), with instability being in the vicinity of 50 to 60°.[20,21]

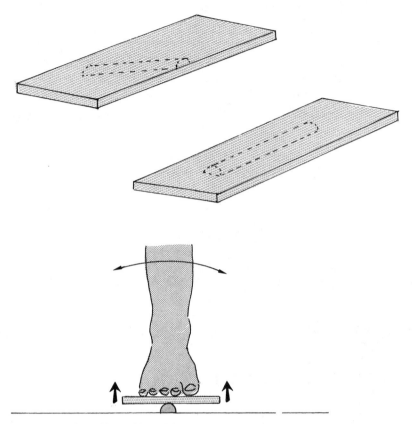

**Figure 8–13.** Tilt and lateral board for proprioceptive training. By changing the angle of the half-round under the board, added proprioceptive training is possible.

In inversion ankle injuries, the extent and site of the ligament injury depend on the position of the foot during the injury. In plantar flexion of the foot, the anterior talofibular ligament is the most vulnerable, whereas in a dorsiflexed foot, the calcaneofibular ligament is the most vulnerable.[22]

In the plantar-flexed foot-ankle injury, inversion produces medial subtalar dislocation. The calcaneofibular ligament sustains tearing, as does the talonavicular ligament and capsule. The sustentaculum tali acts as a fulcrum, allowing the head of the talus to dislocate laterally while the calcaneus moves medially, tearing the lateral talocalcaneal ligament, the capsule, and the calcaneofibular ligament.

## EVERSION SPRAINS

In an injury that forcefully everts the foot, the deltoid ligament sustains the injury (Fig. 8–16). The medial ligament rarely is torn alone. The medial ligament is so strong that avulsion fracture of the tibia frequently occurs.

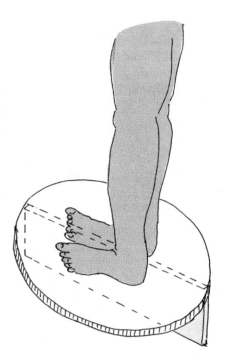

**Figure 8–14.** Tilt board for proprioceptive training. In attempting to balance
while standing on a board placed on a
half-round, the person retrains proprioception.

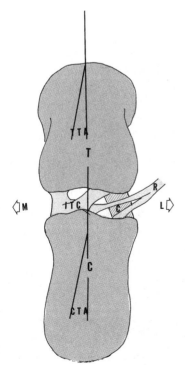

**Figure 8–15.** The ligaments of the talocalcaneal
joint: tibiotalar angle and calcaneotalar angle. The
ligaments of the talocalcaneal joint are shown: ITC
= interosseous talocalcaneal ligament; C = cervical
ligament; and R = the retinacula. M is medial and
L lateral. A line drawn through the tibia and then
the talus (T) forms the tibiotalar angle (TTA), and
a line drawn through the talus and the calcaneus
forms the tibiocalcaneal angle (CTA). An increase
in either of these angles indicates tibiotalar-cal-
caneal instability.

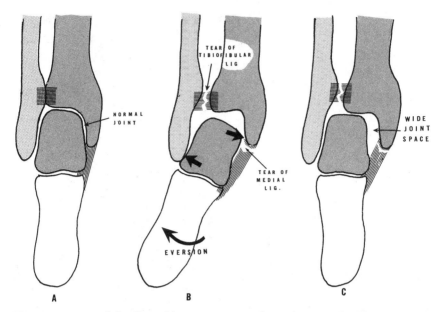

**Figure 8–16.** Medial collateral ligament tear. *A* shows the normal ankle and its ligaments; *B*, a severe eversion injury (curved arrow) causing a talar tilt (straight arrows) and tears of the interosseous and medial ligaments; *C*, the result is widening of the ankle mortise when the ligaments are torn.

A total dislocation of the talus can result. There have been few studies correlating cadaveric studies with clinical studies, so that the significance of this injury has not been fully appreciated.

Stress tomographies have proved effective, whereas routine radiologic studies have not.[23] In an ankle that remains unstable after intensive appropriate rehabilitation, the status of the talocalcaneal joint must be evaluated and treated (Fig. 8–17).

## OSTEOARTHRITIS OF THE ANKLE

Posttraumatic osteoarthritis occurs in the ankle. Several stages have been postulated:[24]

Stage 1: No joint-space narrowing. Early sclerosis and osteophytes.

Stage 2: Narrowing of joint space medially.

Stage 3: Obliteration of the joint space with subchondral bone contact.

Stage 4: Obliteration of the whole joint with complete bone contact.

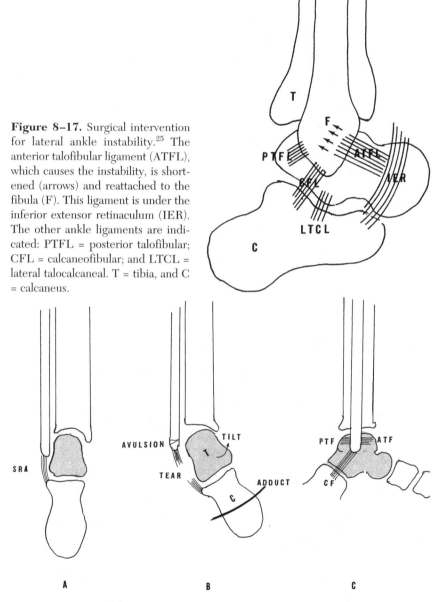

**Figure 8–17.** Surgical intervention for lateral ankle instability.[25] The anterior talofibular ligament (ATFL), which causes the instability, is shortened (arrows) and reattached to the fibula (F). This ligament is under the inferior extensor retinaculum (IER). The other ankle ligaments are indicated: PTFL = posterior talofibular; CFL = calcaneofibular; and LTCL = lateral talocalcaneal. T = tibia, and C = calcaneus.

**Figure 8–18.** Lateral ligamentous sprain and avulsion. (*C*) This depicts the lateral ligaments: PTF = posterior talofibular; ATF = anterior talofibular; and CF = calcaneofibular. (*A*) This is a simple sprain in which the ligaments remain intact and the talus remains stable. (*B*) This depicts a severe adduction of the foot with possible avulsion of the distal fibula, tear of the lateral ligaments, a talar tilt, and even separation of the tibiofibular ligaments.

Osteotomy changes the relationship of the weight-bearing aspects within the ankle joint and merits consideration.

## FRACTURES AND FRACTURE-DISLOCATIONS

Treatment of fractures and fracture-dislocations is beyond the scope of this text, but because these occur from stresses similar to those causing ligament injuries, a careful radiologic study is imperative in severe ankle injuries (Fig. 8–18).

Management requires recognition followed by careful handling in an attempt to gently reduce the gross deformity of the fracture into proper alignment. Splinting in that position, with leg elevation, application of ice, and compression dressing to minimize edema and microhemorrhage, is indicated.

## REFERENCES

1. Machlum, S, and Daljord, OA: Acute sports injuries in Oslo: A one year study. Br J Sports Med 18:181–185, 1984.
2. Garrick, JG: The frequency of injury, mechanism of injury, and epidemiology of ankle sprains. Am J Sports Med 5:241–242, 1977.
3. Lassiter, TE, Malone, TR, and Garrett, WE: Injury to the lateral ligaments of the ankle. Orthop Clin North Am 20(4):629–640, 1989.
4. Bostrom, L: Sprained ankles. I: Anatomic lesions in recent sprains. Acta Chir Scand 128:483–495, 1964.
5. McConkey, JP: Ankle sprains, consequences and mimics. Med Sports Sci 23:39–55, 1987.
6. Hoogenband, CR, Moppes, FI, and Stapert, JW: Clinical diagnosis, arthrography, stress examination and surgical girding after inversion trauma of the ankle. Arch Orthop Trauma Surg 103:115–119, 1984.
7. Johnson, EE, and Markolf, KL: The contribution of the anterior talofibular ligament to ankle laxity. J Bone Joint Surg 65A:81–88, 1983.
8. Watson-Jones, SR: Fractures and Joint Injuries. Livingstone, Edinburgh, 1953.
9. Jackson, DW, Ashley, RD, and Powell, JW: Ankle sprains in young athletes. Clin Orthop 101:201–214, 1974.
10. Brand, RL, Collins, MD, and Tempelton, T: Surgical repair of ruptured lateral ankle ligaments. Am J Sports Med 9:40–44, 1981.
11. Clayton, ML, Miles, JS, and Abdulla, M: Experimental investigations of ligamentous healing. Clin Orthop 140:37–41, 1979.
12. Tillman, LJ, and Cummings, GS: Biological mechanisms of connective tissue mutability, Chap. 1. In Currier, DP, and Nelson, RM (eds): Dynamics of Human Biological Tissues, FA Davis, Philadelphia, 1992, pp 1–44.
13. Cummings, GS, and Tillman, LJ: Remodeling of dense connective tissue in normal adult tissues, Chap. 2. In Currier, DP, and Nelson, RM (eds): Dynamics of Human Biological Tissues. FA Davis, Philadelphia, 1992, pp 45–73.
14. Harrington, KD: Degenerative arthritis of the ankle secondary to long-standing lateral ligament instability. J Bone Joint Surg 61A:354–361, 1979.

15. Freeman, MAR, Dean, MRE, and Hanham, IEF: The etiology and prevention of functional instability of the foot. J Bone Joint Surg 47B:661–668, 1965.
16. Sjolander, P, et al: Can receptors in the collateral ligaments contribute to knee joint stability and proprioception via effects on the fusiform-muscle-spindle system? Neuro–Orthoped 15:65–80, 1994.
17. Johansson, H, Lorentzon, R, Sjolander, P, and Sojka, P: The anterior cruciate ligament. Neuro-Orthoped 9:1–23, 1990.
18. Johansson, H, Sjolander, P, and Sojka, P: Receptors in the knee joint ligaments and their role in the biomechanics of the joint. Crit Rev Biomed Eng 18(5):341–368, 1991.
19. Johansson, H, Sjolander, P, and Sojka, P: Fusiform reflexes in triceps surae muscle elicited by natural and electrical stimulation of joint afferents. Neuro–Orthop 6:67–80, 1988.
20. Brandigan, JW, Pedegana, LR, and Lippert, FG: Instability of the subtalar joint: Diagnosis by stress tomography in three cases. J Bone Joint Surg 59A:321–324, 1977.
21. Chrisman, OD, and Snook, GA: Reconstruction of lateral ligament tears of the ankle: An experimental study and clinical evaluation of seven patients treated by a new modification of the Elmslie procedure. J Bone Joint Surg 51A:904–912, 1969.
22. Clanton, TO: Instability of the subtalar joint. Orthop Clin North Am 20(4): 583–592, 1989.
23. Rubin, G, and Witten, M: The subtalar joint and the symptom of turning over on the ankle: A new method of evaluation utilizing tomography. Am J Orthop 4:16–19, 1962.
24. Takakura, Y, Tanaka, Y, Kumal, T, and Tamai, S: Low tibial osteotomy for osteoarthritis of the ankle. J Bone Joint Surg 77B(1):50–54, 1995.
25. Liu, SH, and Jacobson, KE: A new operation for chronic lateral ankle instability. J Bone Joint Surg 77B(1):55–59, 1995.

# CHAPTER 9

# Neurologic Disorders
# of the Foot

Foot disturbances attributable to nerve involvement usually have intrinsic causes in the foot itself involving "entrapment syndromes." Some neurologic foot problems occur from nervous system impairment located centrally in the brain, spinal cord, or peripheral nerves.

## INNERVATION OF THE FOOT

The foot and ankle are innervated by spinal segments of the L4, L5, S1, and S2 nerve roots (Fig. 9–1). These segments descend the posterior thigh in the sciatic nerve, which ultimately divides into the tibial and peroneal nerves (see Figs. 1–43 through 1–47 in Chap. 1). These nerves supply the muscles of the foot and subserve the sensation of the foot and lower leg.

In the clinical setting, determining the level of a nerve injury with motor deficit requires discerning whether the lesion is at (1) the anterior horn cell level, (2) the nerve root level (Fig. 9–1), or (3) the peripheral nerve level. Sensory impairment also requires determining where along the nerve pattern there is entrapment or disruption.

Nerve identification and localization is done clinically by manual muscle testing, sensory pattern testing, and electrodiagnostic testing.

Nerve function may be impaired by mechanical pressure (entrapment), severance, or intrinsic nerve pathology from numerous sources. Nerves, from their origin in the spinal cord to their effector organ, are at risk for compression and damage with resulting impairment as they pass through bony, fibrous, osteofibrous, or fibromuscular tunnels[1] on the way to their end

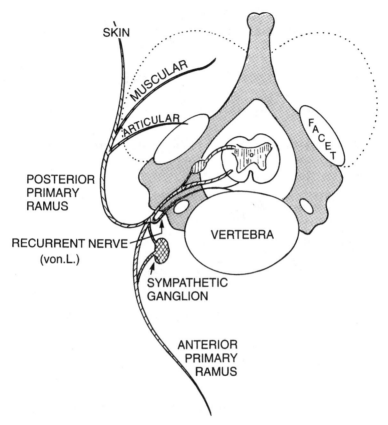

**Figure 9–1.** Formation of a peripheral nerve. The nerves that emerge from the spinal cord are both sensory and motor and converge outside the foramen. They divide into posterior and anterior primary rami. The recurrent nerve returns to the cord carrying sympathetic fibers.

organ. Virtually all nerves carry afferent and efferent impulses with either sensory, motor, or autonomic—usually all three. Clinically testing the end-organ function determines which of these nerve components has the major involvement.

Before describing the specific nerve entrapments, the terms tunnel and canal must be clarified. They are used interchangeably. *Canal,* also termed *tunnel,* implies an enclosed passage composed of either bone or soft tissue.

Nerve compression causes symptoms ranging from sensory deficit to motor loss. The type of sensation shows precisely which nerve is involved. By its character, pain as described by the patient also indicates whether a somatic or a sympathetic nerve is involved (Table 9–1).[2]

Nerve lesions differ as to the degree of injury and its severity (Table 9–2).

Table 9–1

| Nerve Type | Characteristic |
|---|---|
| Sensory (afferent) | Hypalgesia; hypesthesia; sharp quality; loss of discrimination |
| Autonomic | Burning paresthesia; vasomotor disturbances |
| Motor | Fatigue; weakness; loss of function; atrophy; loss of tendon reflex |

In testing an extremity for sensory loss, the following clinical tests are used:

Light touch: brush, cotton, finger

Pain: needle, pin, Tinel test

Temperature: hot or cold water in test tube

Vibration: tuning fork

Two-point discrimination calipers

Sweating: visual chemical tests[3,4]

The dermatomal patterns of the lower extremity and hence the foot and ankle involve the lumbar and sacral roots (Fig. 9–2).

All motor nerve roots in the lower extremity originate from the L4, L5, S1, and S2 roots. Their motor end organs are classified as shown in Fig. 9–3.

## SPINAL PARESIS ORIGIN

*Entrapment*, or injury to a nerve root at the spinal level, may occur at the nerve's emergence from the cord at the intervertebral foramen (Fig. 9–4). To involve the foot and ankle, injury or compression at the spinal level must originate at the L4-5, L5-S1, or S1-S2 levels. This requires a comprehensive exami-

Table 9–2

| Nerve Lesion | Definition |
|---|---|
| Neuropraxia | Temporary loss of function; sensory or motor; no permanent neural disruption |
| Axonotmesis | Disruption of the axons; sheath preserved; recovery dependent on distance from disruption to end organ |
| Neurotmesis | Complete anatomic interruption; complete loss of function; no spontaneous recovery |

Source:   Modified from Pecina, MM, Krompotic-Nemanic, J, and Matkiewitz, AD: Tunnel Syndromes. CRC Press, Boca Raton, FL, 1991.

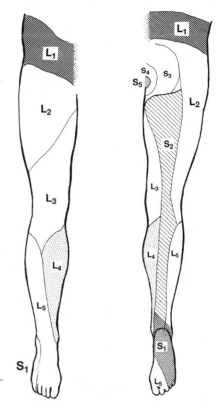

**Figure 9–2.** Dermatomal mapping of lumbar and sacral roots.

nation of the lumbosacral spine[5] with confirmatory testings such as computerized tomography (CT) scanning, magnetic resonance imaging (MRI), myelography, or possibly neurodiagnostic studies such as electromyogram or cortical evoked potentials. Lesions responsible for entrapping the nerve roots to the foot may be caused by disk herniation, foraminal stenosis, tumor, or spondylolisthesis. Careful diagnostic studies are needed to differentiate among these causes. The foot symptoms and signs may be the initial symptoms and signs that ultimately designate the lumbosacral spine as the site of the pathology.

## SCIATIC NERVE

The sciatic nerve is formed in the posterior region of the pelvis from the sacral plexus (Fig. 9–5) derived from the L4, L5, S1, and S2 nerve roots. As these roots merge, they descend through the pelvis at the sacral notch (Fig. 9–6). There they pass under or through the pyriformis muscle, which is innervated via a small branch of the peroneal trunk. In the sciatic nerve's passage, it

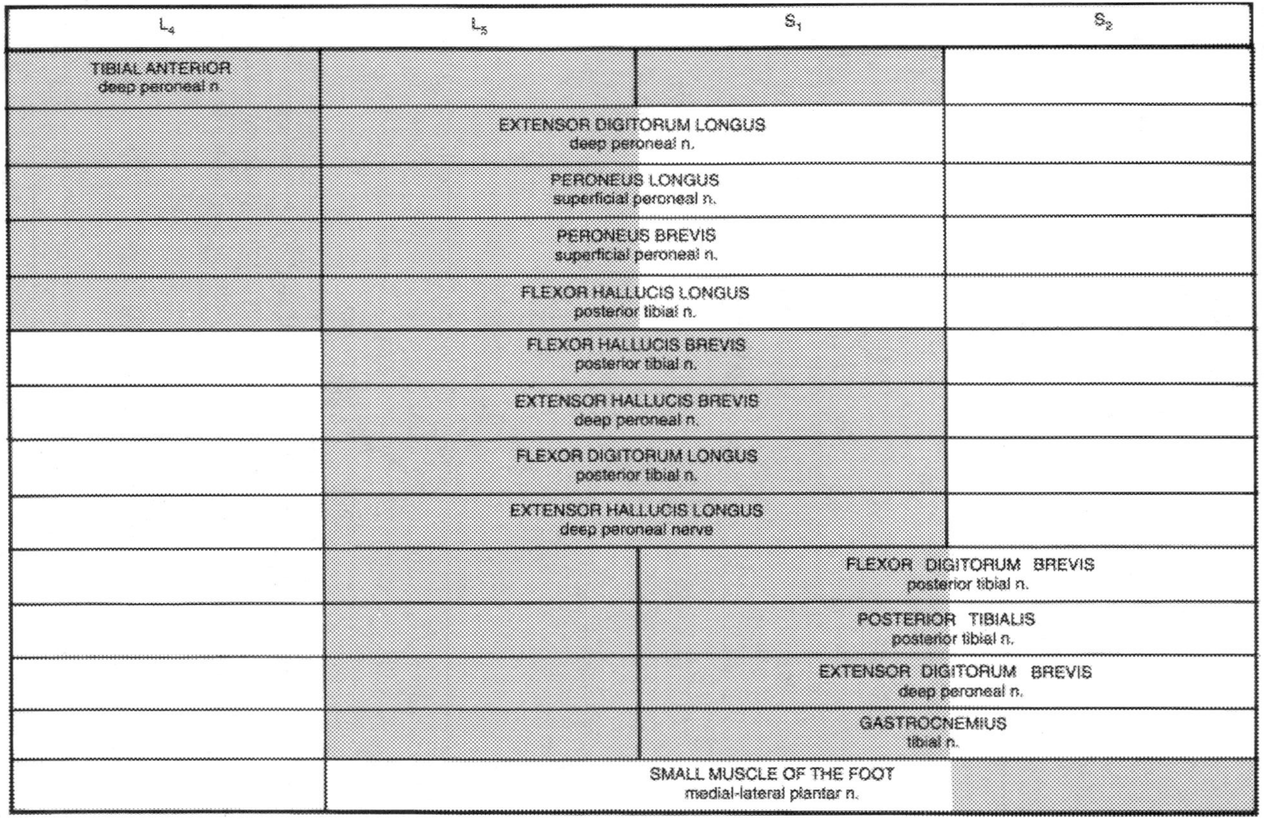

**Figure 9–3.** Origin of nerve roots in spinal segments. Chart shows innervation of the muscles involved in gait. The gray area depicts the spinal segments of the nerve and muscles involved.

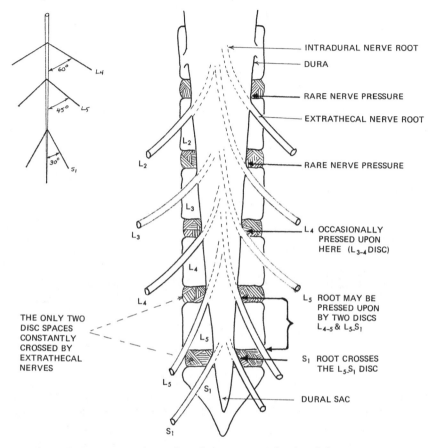

**Figure 9–4.** Relationship of nerve roots to lumbar disk spaces.

innervates motor and sensory fibers to the hamstring muscles, a portion of the adductor magnus, and all the muscles of the leg and foot.

Direct trauma to the sciatic nerve is rare since it is protected by the usual massive gluteal musculature. This is fortunate since a severe lesion of the upper sciatic nerve would result in a flail leg and foot.[6]

## Treatment

Relief of neuropathy pain and paresis of the sciatic nerve includes increasing the space through which the nerve passes and treating the inflammation with the usual modalities and anti-inflammatory medication. Conservative mea-

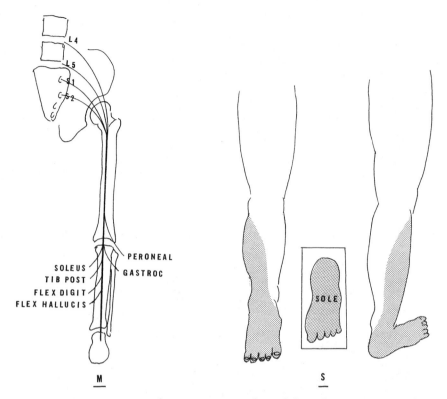

**Figure 9–5.** Sciatic nerve. The sciatic nerve is formed from the L4, L5, S1, and S2 nerve roots. It leaves the pelvis and descends through the sciatic notch down the posterior thigh and leg. It has a motor (M) distribution to the muscles indicated. Its sensory (S) distribution is to the lateral and posterior portion of the foot and the entire plantar surface (sole).

sures, however, rarely afford significant recovery, and operative neurolysis may be necessary.

## SAPHENOUS NERVE

The saphenous nerve is is the termination of the femoral nerve (L2, L3, and L4 roots). After emerging from the femoral triangle, it enters Hunter's canal (subsartorial canal), where it divides into two branches, one of which accompanies the long saphenous vein down the lower leg. In its course, it supplies sensation to the medial knee area and to the medial side of the leg to the foot (Fig. 9–7).

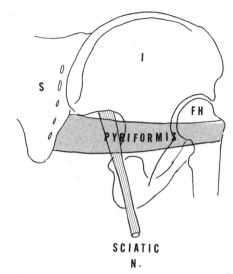

**Figure 9–6.** Sciatic notch. The sciatic nerve emerges from lumbosacral origin in roots L4, L5, S1, and S2 and descends through the sciatic notch. As it descends, it is covered by the pyriformis muscle. I = the ischium; S = the sacrum; FH = the femoral head.

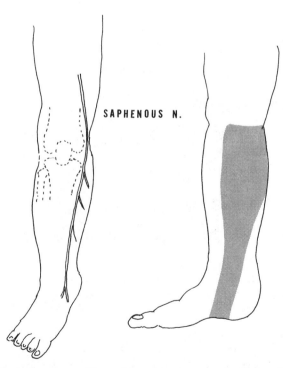

**Figure 9–7.** Saphenous nerve. The saphenous nerve is a continuation of the femoral. It passes the knee medially, where it may be injured in meniscal knee problems. It has primarily a sensory distribution in the lower leg.

A neuropathy of the saphenous nerve is usually manifested as pain. Pain occurs at the knee and radiates downward to the medial aspect of the foot. Causes include vascular obstruction or trauma to the knee joint with a meniscal injury.

## Treatment

If not too severe, rest, modalities, and anti-inflammatory medication may be beneficial. Surgical intervention of any perceived compression at Hunter's canal is indicated.[8,9] Deep knee bends are the usual causative actions and must be avoided or minimized.

## COMMON PERONEAL NERVE

The peroneal nerve is a bifurcation of the sciatic nerve in the posterior aspect of the lower thigh. It travels down the lateral aspect of the popliteal fossa and passes between the biceps femoral tendon and the lateral head of the gastrocnemius (Fig. 9–8).

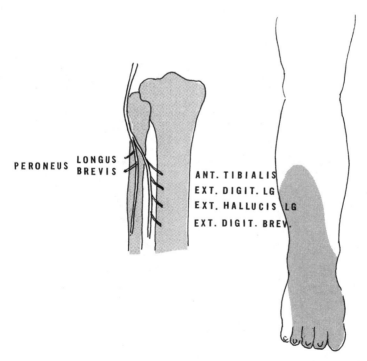

PERONEUS LONGUS BREVIS

ANT. TIBIALIS
EXT. DIGIT. LG
EXT. HALLUCIS LG
EXT. DIGIT. BREV.

**Figure 9–8.** Common peroneal nerve. The motor and sensory distribution of the common peroneal nerve is shown.

The common peroneal nerve supplies the dorsiflexors of the foot-ankle, the evertors of the foot, and sensation from the knee, ankle, and small joints of the foot.[6]

Neuropathy of the common peroneal nerve causes pain in the lateral surface of the leg and foot. Autonomic manifestations are also frequent. There is also weakness of the dorsiflexors and evertors of the foot with atrophy of these muscles. A common cause of this neuropathy is injury to the knee area and the fibular head. Clinically, the patient demonstates a "drop foot."

## Treatment

Corrective shoes with a lateral sole wedge and flare to evert the foot allegedly relax the tension on the peroneal musculature and thus the nerve. Surgical release of the common peroneal nerve at the fibular neck is usually required if conservative measures fail. This is accomplished with simultaneous neurolysis.[10,11]

## SUPERFICIAL PERONEAL NERVE

The superficial peroneal nerve is a division of the common peroneal nerve. The distal lateral nerve separates into two branches that pierce the fascia to innervate the distal lateral position of the leg, dorsum of the foot, and the first four toes other than the web between the big toe and the medial aspect of the second toe (Fig. 9–9).

Pain that is felt is usually burning and superficial with objective hypalgesia and hypesthesia on examination. At the sites of fascial emergence, nodularity is often palpable.

The site not innervated at the web of the dorsum of the foot between the big toe and second toe is innervated by the deep peroneal nerve.[6] Because this nerve is very superficial, it is exposed to trauma. It is also a motor nerve to the extensor digitorum brevis and the first dorsal interosseous muscles.

## Treatment

Conservative measures usually fail to afford relief, even if the offending activities can be completely eliminated. A decompression by fasciotomy has been reported to be effective.[12]

## POSTERIOR TIBIAL NERVE

The posterior tibial nerve usually branches below the lacinate ligament in what is termed the tarsal tunnel (Fig. 9–10), a fibro-osseous tunnel.[13–15] The tarsal tunnel has bony walls consisting of a bony sulcus on the medial side of the calcaneus, posterior process of the talus, and the medial malleolus. It is covered

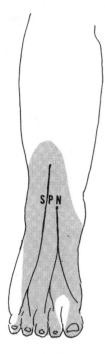

**Figure 9–9.** Superficial peroneal nerve. The motor and sensory distribution of the superficial peroneal nerve is shown as are the sites of emergence through the fascia of the leg.

by the lacinate ligament, which extends between the medial malleolus and the calcaneal tuberosity.

Before entering the tarsal tunnel, the tibial nerve sends a branch that supplies the sensation of the skin of the heel. Compression of the nerve above the ligament may cause heel pain, but heel pain can also be caused by compression of the lateral plantar nerve.

## Treatment

Removing the compression usually suffices. Rest, avoidance of trauma, immobilization possibly with a plaster cast, orthotics, anti-inflammatory medication, and local corticosteroid injections constitute conservative care.[15] In the event that conservative measures indicate surgical intervention, sectioning the superficial layer of the lacinate ligament is not enough. The deep layer must be sectioned, yet preserved, since it is the origin of the abductor hallucis muscle, which is a foot stabilizer.[16,17]

## ANTERIOR TIBIAL NERVE

The anterior tibial nerve is also termed the deep peroneal nerve and the musculoskeletal nerve.[6] Compression syndromes of the nerve, termed *anterior*

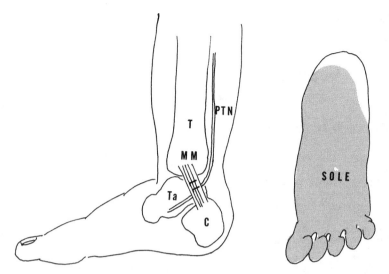

**Figure 9–10.** Posterior tibial nerve. The posterior tibial nerve passes under the lacinate ligament (LL) into the foot in what is termed the tarsal tunnel. This ligament connects the calcaneus (C) with the medial malleolus (MM), which is at the terminus of the tibia (T). It passes over the talus (Ta). On leaving the tunnel, it divides into three branches (medial plantar, lateral plantar, and calcaneal). It supplies sensation to the skin of the plantar surface of the foot (sole) and supplies the intrinsic muscles of the foot.

*tarsal tunnel syndrome* (Fig. 9–11), have been described in runners, skiers, and dancers.[18,19] Injuries have included repetitive ankle sprains from wearing tight-heeled shoes or ski boots.[20–22]

The nerve becomes superficial below the cruciate crural ligament and is poorly covered. Because it directly overlies the tarsal bones, it is subject to direct trauma.

Diagnosis is suggested by localized pain and tenderness with anesthesia over the area at the cleft of the first and second toes. If the motor branch is affected, there can be atrophy of the muscle mass of the short extensors and weakness noted on toe extension. Forced plantar flexion of the foot and toes aggravates the pain, as will direct pressure. Perineural injection of an anesthetic agent is diagnostic and also therapeutic.

## Treatment

Rest, removal of the offending pressure, anti-inflammatory medication, and local analgesic and steroid injection are usually effective. Surgical intervention must ascertain that the overlying extensor retinaculum is adequately resected. There is also the possibility that adhesions with the extensor tendons are offenders.

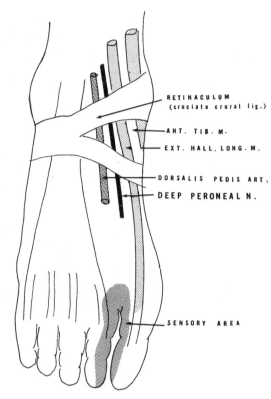

RETINACULUM
(cruciate crural lig.)

ANT. TIB. M.

EXT. HALL. LONG. M.

DORSALIS PEDIS ART.

DEEP PERONEAL N.

SENSORY AREA

**Figure 9–11.** Deep peroneal nerve: Anterior tarsal tunnel syndrome. The deep peroneal nerve becomes superficial as it emerges below the cruciate crural ligament. There it is vulnerable to trauma, causing pain and numbness in the shaded area shown in the figure.

## INTERDIGITAL NEUROPATHIES

The interdigital nerves, also termed the common digital nerves, are a frequent source of metatarsal head pain. The interdigital nerves are sensory to the toes and are a prolongation of the medial and lateral plantar nerves. In their passage, they pass within compartments (Fig. 9–12).

In their passage, these nerves change course over and against the deep transverse tarsal ligament that binds the metatarsal heads together. This angulation is most marked when the toes are hyperextended and the metatarsophalangeal (MP) joints (Fig. 9–13) flexed. MP flexion relieves the pressure on the interdigital nerve(s). Direct downward pressure on the nerve is also possible. Pressure is greater in a foot with fixed, hyperextended MP joints from other causes such as a herniated lumbar disk, spastic paresis, and so on.

Diagnosis is that of localized pain and tenderness with some causalgic signs and symptoms often being associated. Direct digital pressure between the metatarsal heads differentiates pain from metatarsalgia (see Chap. 5, Fig. 5–34).

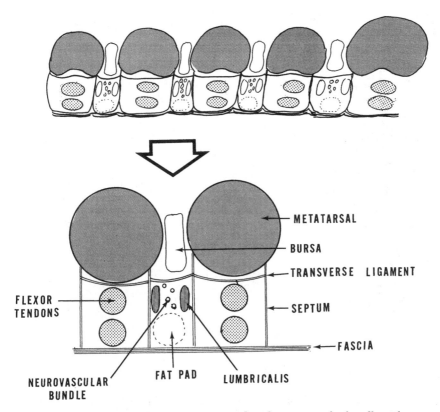

**Figure 9–12.** Compartments containing interdigital neurovascular bundles. The contents of the interdigital compartments are depicted.

## Treatment

The most important measure is to decrease the mechanism of interdigital pressure: low-heel shoes with broad forefoot, avoidance of toe stance, correction of hyperextended toes and their cause. Pressure pads afford relief of pressure. Interdigital injection of analgesic agents and steroids affords temporary relief. If neuromata are suspected, surgical excision is indicated.

## MORTON'S NEUROMA

Morton's neuroma is entrapment of an interdigital nerve that results in a fusiform swelling of the digital nerve. It is most commonly found where the interdigital nerve branches into the contiguous aspects of the digits (Fig. 9–14). It is usually found between the third and fourth toes and unusually between the second and third metatarsals.

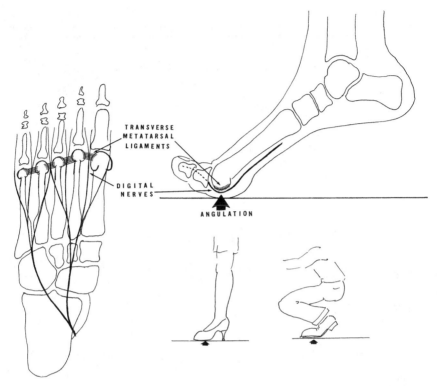

**Figure 9–13.** Entrapment of an interdigital nerve. The interdigital nerves originate from the plantar nerves in the sole of the foot and pass between the transverse metatarsal ligaments to supply sensation to the toes. If they become angulated at the ligaments because of abnormal posture or activities, they cause pain and numbness in the toes.

# FLACCID PARESIS

A neurologic lower-extremity problem that affects the foot is flaccid paresis. Causes include poliomyelitis, Guillain-Barré syndrome, sciatic neuritis, herniated lumbar disk, and numerous other systemic neuropathies of which diabetes is a factor (see Chap. 10). The diagnosis is made by means of a clinical history and confirmatory laboratory tests. Usually the condition is a motor deficit rather than a sensory abnormality with pain, although the latter is possible.

If the paresis or paralysis is significant and impairs ambulation, bracing is indicated. These braces vary significantly and are modified by the size of the individual, the degree of the paresis, the precise motor deficit, and the needs of the individual. Several examples are illustrated in Figures 9–15 through 9–18.

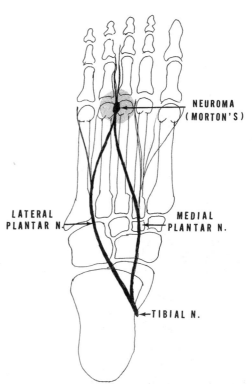

**Figure 9–14.** Morton's interdigital neuroma. Morton's neuroma is a neurofibroma of the interdigital nerve. The most frequent site is the third branch of the medial plantar nerve as it merges with the lateral plantar nerve to form the digital nerve between the third and fourth toes. It more rarely occurs at other interdigital nerve sites. Pain and hypalgesia occurs in the area, and pain can be elicited by digital pressure between the metatarsal heads.

# SPASTIC PARALYSIS

In an upper motor neuron lesion with spasticity, the foot assumes an equinus position, which prevents dorsiflexion during stance and gait. The deep-tendon reflexes are hyperactive, and there is spasticity, clonus, and a diagnostic Babinski sign. It is the spasticity and equinus that impair function. The foot does not clear on the swing-through phase. During the stance phase, the heel does not contact the floor, and when it does, it does so by hyperextending the knee.

Prolonged equinus causes contracture of the gastrocnemius-soleus complex, which defies elongation allowing dorsiflexion.

## Treatment

Treating the spasticity is attempted with medications. Physical therapy passively stretches the Achilles–gastrocnemius-soleus complex actively and with home exercises. Strengthening the anterior tibialis muscle allegedly also causes contralateral relaxation (agonist-antagonist) of the plantar flexors.

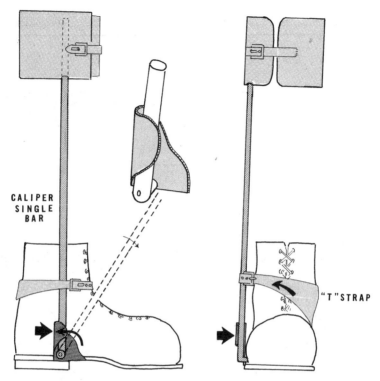

**Figure 9–15.** Short leg brace with a right angle stop. This short leg brace prevents plantar flexion beyond the distance corrected by the brace shown in the center of the illustration. This prevents equinus, and a "T" strap corrects inversion of the spastic foot.

The braces illustrated in Figures 9–15 through 9–17 are also useful in improving the gait and stretching the plantar flexion complexes. Because spasticity also causes varus, a T strap applied to the single-bar, short leg brace is helpful (Fig. 9–19).

## VARUS FOOT IN CEREBRAL PALSY

In cerebral palsy, imbalance of the invertor and evertor muscles results in varus alignment of the foot, with the functional impairment being weight-bearing instability or foot clearance during the swing phase.

Foot mechanics have been analyzed, and the sagittal movements during weight bearing are familiar. The muscular actions in impaired individuals affect mostly the coronal and transverse planes, which occur in the subtalar joints.

At foot strike, the calcaneus falls into valgus and there is medial shear on the subtalar joint, leading to internal rotation of the talus, which increases dur-

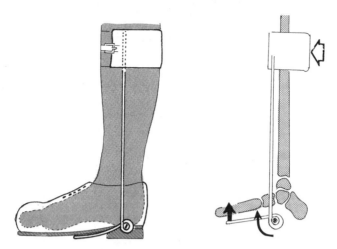

**Figure 9–16.** Piano-wire dorsiflexion brace. When there is minimal contraction of the gastrocnemius-soleus muscle as in a flaccid paresis, a piano-wire brace gives flexible dorsiflexion of the ankle during the swing phase of gait.

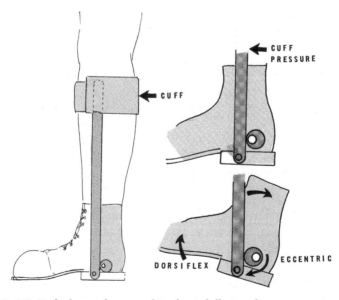

**Figure 9–17.** Night brace that stretches the Achilles tendon–gastrocnemius-soleus complex. The eccentric ankle joint forces the shoe that has a sole bar for inflexibility into dorsiflexion. This passively and constantly stretches the plantar flexor tissues. The degree of dorsiflexion can be modified by rotating the ankle joint. Its main use is as a night brace.

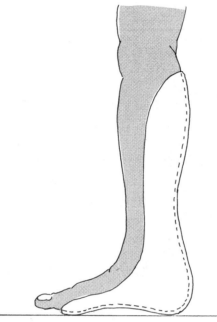

**Figure 9–18.** Plastic posterior molded lower-leg brace. To maintain dorsiflexion during stance and through the swing phase of gait, a molded plastic (fiberglass) brace can be molded to the precise form of the foot and ankle. Corrections at the arch, posterior metatarsal heads, and varus-valgus of the ankle can be incorporated.

ing the stance phase (Fig. 9–20) because of rotation of the tibia. Weight bearing begins at the heel and proceeds along the lateral border of the foot toward the metatarsal heads, with the major propulsive thrust by the distal phalanx (Fig. 9–21).

The posterior compartment muscles influence the mechanics of the foot. As the foot pushes off, it supinates by virtue of the triceps surae, tibialis posterior, flexor hallucis longus, flexor digitorum longus, tibialis anterior, and extensor hallucis longus muscles, of which the anterior tibialis, posterior tibialis, and triceps surae muscles are the most important.[23]

The tibialis anterior muscle dorsiflexes and supinates the foot, while the posterior tibialis muscle inverts (adducts) and plantar flexes. The anterior tibialis is primarily active during the swing phase of gait, and the posterior and triceps surae during stance phase.

The extensor digitorum longus, peroneus longus, and peroneus brevis muscles are *evertors*. The extensor digitorum longus acts with the anterior tibialis during swing phase and prevents, or minimizes, supination and inversion.

Gait analysis of the cerebral palsied is inconclusive with abnormalities of both the tibialis anterior and the tibialis posterior identified as being hyperactive. At the onset of swing phase, if the anterior tibialis becomes overly active

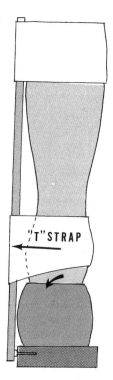

"T" STRAP

**Figure 9–19.** T strap attached to short leg brace to correct valgus. When there is a severe valgus condition and the leg requires a short leg brace, a T strap can be applied to the brace bar on the inside of the leg, which pulls (straight arrow) the leg-ankle into varus (curved arrow).

and the posterior tibialis inactive, this is an indication for surgical intervention (tendon transplant) of the anterior tibialis.

Overactivity of the tibialis posterior interferes with the stance phase, contributing to equinus and deficient lateral shear. It is important to determine whether the foot varus occurs in the swing or the stance phase—or both. This finding, which determines which surgical procedure merits consideration, can be determined by foot pressure studies and simultaneous EMG studies.[24–27]

Unfortunately, the above studies do not clearly distinguish between the motions of the forefoot and the hindfoot.

Broadly speaking, cerebral palsy is a neurologic deficit resulting from cerebral dysfunction acquired during the gestation, parturition, or neonatal period. Functionally, it runs the gamut of neurologic, orthopedic, and psychologic problems.[28] The foot of the cerebral palsied therefore also runs this gamut; only the spastic equinovarus foot has been discussed.

## Treatment

Initially in treating the ambulation problems in cerebral palsy, the child is often fitted with a double-long leg brace with a pelvic band or a Knight spiral

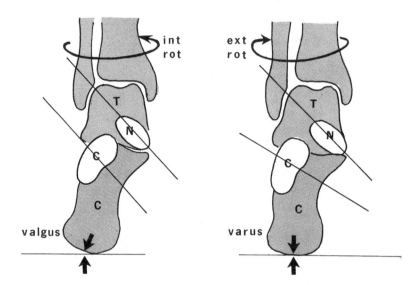

**Figure 9–20.** Supination of the foot during rotation of the leg. In the weight-bearing stance, internal rotation causes valgus of the foot with pronation (*left* figure). During weight bearing in the stance phase, external rotation (*right* figure) causes the foot to rotate at the subtalar joint and supinate the foot for the ultimate swing-through phase. T denotes the talus and C the calcaneus with their facets designated N (navicular) and C (cuboid).

brace with ring locks at the hips and knees and a 90° stop at the ankles. Physical therapy exercises done passively *to* the patient and ultimately *by* the patient are initiated and modified. Braces are also moderated with the needs presented. It is hoped that adequate and persistent physical therapy and bracing will delay or deny the need for surgical intervention. The surgical techniques used are beyond the scope of this text,[29,30] but should be the decision of the consulting orthopedic surgeon.

Recently, medical opinions have changed in the management of spasticity. Visual evaluation of the spastic gait fails to determine the extent and effect of spasticity and/or weakness of specific muscles, which causes difficulty in determining the efficacy of tenotomies or nerve-block procedures.

With newer techniques of weight-bearing pressure plate analysis and simultaneous electromyographic studies during all phases of the gait, this conclusion permits a more scientific basis for therapeutic procedures. Phenol nerve blocks or botulism toxoid injection into specific muscle groups enhances the possibility of long-duration benefit.

Multidiscipline management of spasticity is thus needed but is more effective when it combines anesthesiologic intervention using nerve blocks and botulism toxoid after a meaningful evaluation from podiatrists and physiatrists

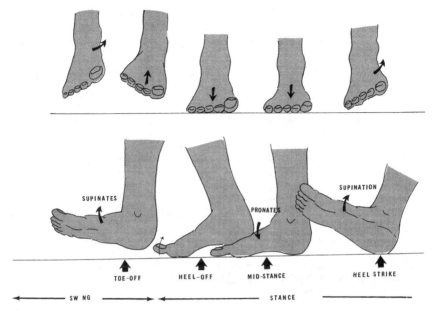

**Figure 9–21.** Foot and ankle aspect of gait. In normal gait, the foot dorsiflexes and supinates during the toe-off and heel-strike phase. It is pronated at heel off and mid-stance phase. With spasticity or flaccidity, all these aspects are altered and must be evaluated and corrected.

skilled in pressure plate and electromyographic evaluation techniques. Ultimately, physical therapy, orthopedic surgical intervention, and orthotists, as well as neurologic and pediatric testing, complete the rehabilitation team.

# REFERENCES

1. Pecina, MM, Krompotic-Nemanic, J, and Markiewitz, AD: Tunnel Syndromes, CRC Press, Boca Raton, 1991.
2. Cailliet, R: Pain: Mechanisms and Management. FA Davis, Philadelphia 1993.
3. Gutmann, L: Atypical deep peroneal neuropathy. J Neurol Neurosurg Psychiatry 33:453–456, 1970.
4. McElvenny, RT: Etiology and surgical treatment of intractable pain about fourth metatarsophalangeal joint. J Bone Joint Surg 25:675–679, 1943.
5. Cailliet, R: Low Back Pain Syndromes, ed 5., FA Davis, Philadelphia, 1994.
6. Kopell, HP, and Thompson, WAL: Sciatic Nerve, Sciatic Notch, Chapter 10, In Kopell, HP, and Thompson, WAL: Peripheral Entrapment Neuropathies, Williams & Wilkins, Baltimore, 1963, pp. 55–58.
7. Haymaker, W, and Woodhall, B: Injuries of the Peripheral Nerves Derived from the Lumbar Plexus. In Haymaker, W, and Woodhall, B: Peripheral Nerve Injuries, ed 2. WB Saunders, Philadelphia, 1953, pp 282–285.

8. Worth, RM, et al: Saphenous nerve entrapment: A cause of medial knee pain. Am J Sports Med 12:80, 1984.

9. Dumitru, D, and Windsor, RE: Subsartorial entrapment of the saphenous nerve of a competitive female body builder. Phys Sportsmed 17:116, 1989.

10. Moller, BN, and Kadin, S: Entrapment of the common peroneal nerve. Am J Sports Med 15:90, 1987.

11. Leach, RE, Purnell, MB, and Saito, A: Peroneal nerve entrapment in runners. Am J Sports Med 17:287, 1989.

12. Styf, J: Entrapment of the superficial peroneal nerve: Diagnosis and results of decompression. J Bone Joint Surg 71B:131, 1989.

13. Keck, Ch: Tarsal tunnel syndrome. J Bone Joint Surg 44A:180, 1962.

14. Lam, SJS: Tarsal tunnel compression of nerve contents. Lancet 2:1354, 1962.

15. Lam, SJS: Posterior nerve entrapment. J Bone Joint Surg 49B:87, 1967.

16. Androic, S: Reumatizam 14:12, 1967.

17. Edwards, WG, et al: Surgical release of the posterior tibial nerve. JAMA 207:716, 1969.

18. Deese, JM, Jr, and Baxter, DE: Compressive neuropathies of the lower extremities. J Musculoskel Med 5:68, 1988.

19. Schon, LC, and Baxter, DE: Neuropathies of the foot and ankle in athletes. Clin Sports Med 9:489, 1990.

20. Lindenbaum, BI: Ski boot compression syndrome. Clin Orthop 140:19, 1979.

21. Gessini, L, Jandolo, B, and Pietrangeli, A: The anterior tarsal syndrome: Report of four cases. J Bone Joint Surg 66A:786, 1984.

22. Murphy, PC, and Baxter, DE: Nerve entrapment of the foot and ankle in runners. Clin Sports Med 4:753, 1985.

23. Sussman, MD (ed): The Diplegic Child: Evaluation and Management. AAOS Publishers, Rosemont, IL, 1992, pp 389–396.

24. Barto, PS, Supinski, RS, and Skinner, SR: Dynamic EMG findings in the varus hindfoot deformity and spastic cerebral palsy. Day Med Child Neurol 26:88–93, 1984.

25. Wills, CA, Hoffer, MM, and Perry, J: A comparison of foot switch and EMG analysis of varus deformities of the feet of children with cerebral palsy. Dev Med Child Neurol 30:227–231, 1988.

26. Alexander, I, and DeLozier, G: Integrated three-dimensional motion analysis and dynamic foot pressure assessments in the evaluation of foot and ankle mechanics. Presented at Seventh Annual Summer Meeting of the American Orthopaedic Foot and Ankle Society. Boston, MA, July 25–28, 1991.

27. Hoffer, MM, Barakat, G, and Koffman, M: 10-year follow-up of split anterior tibial tendon transfer in cerebral palsied patients with spastic equinovarus deformity. J Ped Orthop 5:432–434, 1985.

28. Rusk, HA: Rehabilitation of patient with cerebral palsy, Chap 26. In Rusk, HA: Rehabilitation Medicine, ed 4. CV Mosby, St Louis, 1977, pp 474–495.

29. Baker, LD: A rational approach to the surgical needs of the cerebral palsy patient. J Bone Joint Surg (Am) 38:313, 1956.

30. Silver, CM, and Simon, SD: Operative treatment of cerebral palsy involving the lower extremity. J Inter Coll Surg 27:457, 1957.

# CHAPTER 10

# Causalgia and Other Reflex Sympathetic Dystrophies

Reflex sympathetic dystrophy occurs so frequently in posttraumatic conditions and yet is so often overlooked by the uninformed, uneducated, and unaware physician that an entire chapter is essential in considering painful conditions of the lower extremity.

Reflex sympathetic dystrophy (RSD) involves the lower extremities somewhat less frequently than it does the upper. This condition was seen more frequently in war times; however, with the increasing incidence of warlike injuries in civilian life, such as contact sports activities and auto and motorcycle accidents, it is increasing in frequency.

From injuries in the vicinity of the knee, the foot, and ankle and their treatment, conservative and surgical, the presence of RSD in the lower extremity may be overlooked. RSD in the absence of causalgia is often misdiagnosed and mistreated with severe disabling sequelae. RSD manifestations resulting from trauma to any part of the lower extremity are usually noted in the foot, ankles, and toes.

The most frequent cause of RSD in the lower extremity is iatrogenic from surgical interventions and tight casts, with injury near, or of, the nerves of the lower extremity.

## REFLEX SYMPATHETIC DYSTROPHY

The condition termed reflex sympathetic dystrophy now encompasses many neuromuscular vasomotor disabling conditions of both the lower and the upper extremities. This condition, aptly termed a syndrome, is known to follow virtually any form of local injury, major or minor. The condition, originally termed *causalgia*, implied "burning pain" with associated neurovascular symp-

243

tomatology. This syndrome may be further broken down into major and minor versions wherein pain, burning or otherwise, need not be associated. By so delineating the condition, it is more apt to be recognized early and properly treated.

Bonica[1] divided RSD into major and minor by means of the following subdivisions:

| Major | Minor |
| --- | --- |
| Causalgia | Shoulder-hand-finger syndrome |
| Thalamic syndrome | Postmyocardial infarct |
| Phantom limb | Postcerebrovascular attack |
| | Postinjection |
| | Postfracture, cast, splint |
| | Post-overuse syndrome: Now termed *repetitive trauma* disorders |

It is apparent from the table that with the minor dystrophies, any trauma can be implicated, which may indicate an incident so minor that the cause is often difficult to remember.

Certainly RSD is a major complication of any extremity impairment, painful or painless; thus, its recognition must be entertained with any complaint of an extremity that is presented by the patient, especially when the patient describes persistent and "atypical" pain.

The literature indicates that *burning pain* and associated symptoms following a peripheral nerve injury was noted by Paré[2] in the sixteenth century. The condition reached prominence during the American Civil War (1864) when it was described by Mitchell and coworkers.[3] Mitchell described the condition in wounded soldiers who developed a "burning pain" following a peripheral nerve injury, usually from gunshot wounds. Mitchell employed the term "causalgia" for describing the burning character of the pain and is credited with originally describing this condition, which is currently classified as a major reflex sympathetic dystrophy.

Many clinicians followed with descriptive discussions of this condition. Letievant[4] of France (1873) described the condition as neurologic in causation. Sudeck[5] (1900) published a classic description of the radiologic characteristics of bone osteoporosis following trauma with subsequent RSD. Leriche[6] (1916) described the condition as a sequela of the sympathetic nervous system, which led to the use of peripheral sympathectomy as a favored and successful treatment of RSD. Then RSD was largely forgotten until World War II, when numerous cases were reported and the clinical condition revived.

Numerous terms have been used in the literature. These include algodystrophy, sympathalgia, neurovascular reflex sympathetic dystrophy, traumatic angiospasm, traumatic vasospasm, Sudeck atrophy, posttramatic osteoporosis, posttraumatic painful osteoporosis, shoulder-hand-finger syndrome, and so on. Pain persists, often after the initial trauma subsides, and pain is considered to remain in the peripheral nerve distribution via sympathetic nerve fibers. This pain has been labeled *sympathetically maintained pain* (SMP). Where there is less evidence of sympathetic nervous system involvement, yet persistence of the pain, the term *sympathetic independent pain* (SID) is used.[7]

All of the above terms allude to the following clinical manifestations:

1. Persistent pain—variously described, but frequently of a "burning" quality, although not necessarily of this specific quality.
2. Vasomotor changes manifested as hyperthermia often followed by coldness.
3. The presence of subcutaneous edema becoming rapidly nonpitting.
4. The presence of sensory changes—at first hyperesthesia and later hypesthesia.
5. Ultimate trophic changes, such as atrophy of the skin, muscle, and bone, causing functional impairment. Ultimate significant osteoporosis. Atrophic osteoarthrosis.[8,9]

Causalgia has been defined by the International Association for the Study of Pain (IASP)[10] as "a syndrome of sustained burning pain after traumatic nerve lesion combined with vasomotor and sudomotor dysfunction and later trophic changes." Amplification of the RSD syndrome now includes many conditions of RSD without "burning pain," yet all with the vasomotor and sudomotor symptoms and findings. This conforms to the SID pain described by Roberts.[7] The basic mechanisms, pathophysiology, and symptoms[11] in any form of RSD are similar enough to justify the diagnostic term and therapies.

Defining each word of the term reflex sympathetic dystrophy clarifies the disease entity. *Dystrophy* indicates wasting of the muscular and bony tissues of the region as well as abnormal growth of the nails of the extremity and hyperkeratosis of the skin. *Sympathetic* indicates vasomotor and sudomotor changes such as inappropriate sweating, coldness, and color changes of the extremity from vasoconstriction or vasodilatation. *Reflex* indicates that the signs emanate from the sympathetic nervous system distribution of the extremity. Another confirming diagnostic fact of RSD is its beneficial response to sympathetic interruption.

Onset of pain varies between major RSD (causalgia) and minor RSD in that the former has either an immediate onset of pain or an onset within at least a brief period of time, whereas minor RSD may have a delay of pain of several days to months. The character of pain is inevitably described as a "burning" sensation, which qualifies the condition as being RSD.

The site of this syndrome is distal in the extremity, whether it is upper—shoulder-hand-finger—or lower—knee-ankle-foot-toes.

The mechanisms involved have been variously postulated. Mitchell[3] proposed the mechanism as being from "an inexplicable reflex in the spinal cord centers felt in remote regions outside the distribution of the wounded nerve." This definition has been modified by the author, but the idea was retained. Numerous concepts have been postulated, but more recently a concept has been offered by Devor[12] in which he suggests that the injury damages or transects (cuts across) the involved nerve.

This appealing theory involves understanding the structure of nerve axons and the theory of axoplasmic transport. The hypothesis is exemplified in Figure 10–1.[13]

Neuronal function is now considered to be axonal transport of protein and other materials needed by the tissues supplied by the nerve. Sensory impulses are also supplied by axonal transport.

The neuron cell body undergoes a high level of protein synthesis, which is conveyed along the length of the nerve fiber. This transport mechanism has been shown to be dependent on an adequate blood supply. Pressure on the

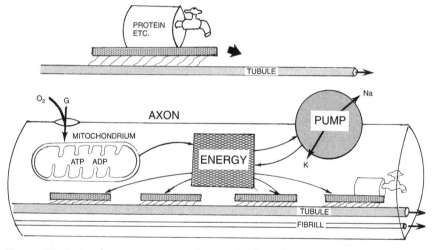

**Figure 10–1.** Axoplasmic transport: A theory. The flow of protein and other derivatives begins with the entry of glucose (G) into the nerve fiber. Glycolysis and phosphorylation occur ($O_2$) in the mitochondria through the metabolism of adenosine triphosphate (ATP), which creates the energy for the sodium pump. This pump regulates the balance between sodium (Na) and potassium (K) and determines the activity of the nerve. The transport filaments (FIBRILL) move along the axon by oscillation and carry the nutritive protein elements along the nerve pathway. (From Cailliet, R: Knee Pain and Disability, ed 3. FA Davis, Philadelphia, 1992, p 228, Fig. 7.13. Data from Ochs, S: Axoplasmic transport—A basis for neural pathology. In Dyke, PJ, Thomas, PK, and Lambert, EH (eds): Peripheral Neuropathy, WB Saunders, Philadelphia, 1975, pp 213–230.)

nerve axon and/or its blood flow will impair axonal transport. The flow via the axon microtubules and neurofilaments is impaired. Variation of the components of the proteins of the peripheral nerve will also determine the end result of axonal impairment.

After a nerve has been constricted the fibers may show collateral branching.[14,15] During recovery of the injured nerve, the exposed regenerating surface of the axon undergoes more than normal accumulation of receptors. These receptors are alpha-adrenogenic, which results in that nerve developing abnormal electrical properties.[16] These excessive, and possibly abnormal, receptors become ectopic pacemakers, which lead to spontaneous depolarization. Because they are numerous and excessive, they bombard the central nervous system and interfere with the normal central processing of sensory information. The central nervous system, which is already in a state of hyperactivity and hyperreceptivity from previous bombardment by unmyelinated nerve fiber impulses, is now more accessible to the persistence of pain because of this added, excessive release of distal epinephrine impulses from these new branchings of the nerve fibers (Fig. 10–2).[12]

The peripheral stimuli originate because of the neurons' abnormal chemosensitivity and mechanosensitivity, not as a result of otherwise physiologic stimuli.

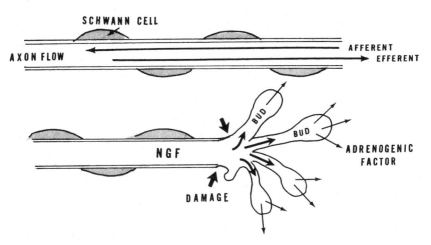

**Figure 10–2.** Axonal outgrowths forming a neuroma (schematic). *Upper* drawing depicts a normal nerve axon flow. After a nerve injury from compression or partial to total severance (*bottom* drawing), the nerve growth factor (NGF) stimulates the nerve to advance distally, forming "buds," which in turn create more nerve endings. By virtue of greater secretion of adrenogenic factors from these additional buds, the nerve becomes more sensitive to adrenogenic agonists and transmits more potential pain fiber impulses to the spinal cord.

Centrally, the aberrant sensory processing from this barrage produces a sensation of pain (paresthesias) and the altered sympathetic reflexes produce the somatic characteristics of RSD (Fig. 10–3).

There are other theories that postulate the involvement of the peripheral nervous system rather than central mechanisms. At the site of the nerve injury, a synapse between efferent sympathetic and afferent pain fibers occurs, which "short-circuits" the sensory information.[17,18] This concept has been refuted because it does not explain why a sympathetic nerve block distal to the lesion is effective. Another peripheral concept invokes liberation at the involved area[6] of algesic substances (nociceptive), which produce local hyperalgesia, which, in turn, produces a sustained, vicious cycle.

Of the numerous central mechanisms postulated, the concept of bombardment of the dorsal horn cells in laminae IV to VI by the peripheral nociceptor substances is widely held (Fig. 10–4).

As stated by Rizzi and coworkers,[19] an unanswered question is why causalgia occurs most often with a "partial" nerve lesion rather than a complete lesion and why there is such a low incidence of causalgia with so many partial nerve lesions.

The psychologic state of the individual at the time of the injury has also been postulated as a significant factor. Much research is still needed to ascertain the neuropsychologic-humeral susceptibility of individuals under extreme anxiety, which predisposes patients having trauma to develop causalgic RSD.

A hypothesis has recently been advanced[20] as to why many cases of RSD occur after a relatively minor trauma or why pain and other somatic symptoms are exacerbated by emotional stress. It is postulated that pre-existing anxiety or stress increases the release of norepinephrine, which increases arteriolar hyperactivity. The effects of vasospasm, ischemia, and nociceptor release on neural tissues already bathed by excessive norepinephrine brought on from the anxiety and stress result in RSD.

The neural-psychologic-humeral aspect of the emotions to pain merits discussion in the section on the sympathetic system, especially because excessive norepinephrine released from anxiety, stress, and fear is considered to play a prominent role.

Psychologic stress over a long period of time causes stimulation of the hypothalamus via the nucleus reticularis paragigantocellularis (RPG) in the medulla. From the medulla, there are many projections to the hypothalamus, especially the paraventricular nuclei (PVN) (Fig. 10–5).[21] The PVNs contain neurons that release vasopressin and oxytocin, which enter the posterior pituitary gland.

There is a chemical interplay between the posterior and anterior pituitary glands with a release of corticotropin hormone and ACTH. This is termed *preponderance* of sympathetic release. The resulting hypothalamic-pituitary-adrenal axis (HPA) is the neurologic-hormonal response to stress.[22–24]

In many painful states, hypersensitivity of the involved tissues is apparently mediated through mechanoreceptors in areas already hypersensitized.

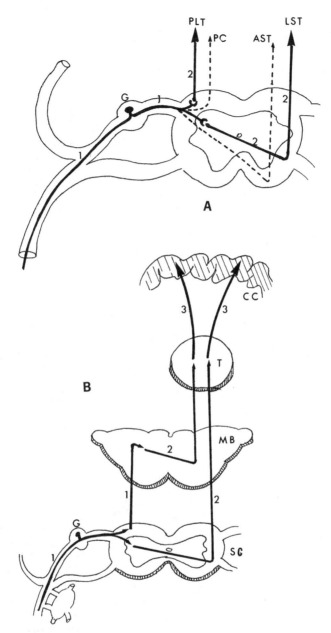

**Figure 10–3.** Neuronal pathways of pain. (*A*) Depicts the course of sensory fibers (1) in a segmental nerve with its ganglia in the dorsal root (G). Upon entrance into the cord, the fibers ascend, on the same side (1) (2), in the posterior lateral tract (PLT) and decussate to cross (2) into the lateral spinothalamic tract via secondary neurons (2). The posterior columns (PC) transmit position sense. Ascending spinal tracts (AST) convey tactile sensation. (*B*) The first-stage neuron (1) to the cord via the ganglion (G) stimulates the second-stage neuron (2) in the midbrain (MB), then into the thalamus (T). The third-stage neuron (3) ascends to the cerebral cortex (CC). These fibers are termed thalamo-cortical pathways.

249

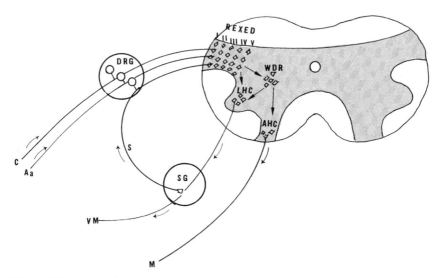

**Figure 10–4.** Causalgic (autonomic) pain transmission pathways. Trauma irritates the endings of somatic afferent (unmyelinated) C fibers, mechanofibers, and autonomic (sympathetic) fibers, causing impulses to proceed to cells of the layers of Rexed (I), (II), (III), (IV), and (V) within the gray matter of the cord. An interneuronal pathway excites the lateral horn cells of the autonomic system, transmitting impulses to the sympathetic ganglion. The impulses from the sympathetic ganglion return to the dorsal root ganglion (dorsal GGL) as sensory impulses. The mechanofibers transmit impulses that transmit allodynia impulses in the circuit.

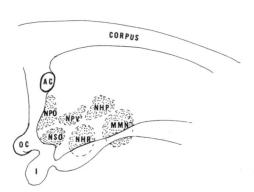

**Figure 10–5.** The principal nuclei of the hypothalamus. There are various groups of hypothalamic nuclei. The efferent impulses that pass through the thalamus via the hypothalamus are probably the major routes to the cerebral cortex. These nuclei are as follows: NVP = nucleus paraventricularis; NPO = nucleus preopticus; NSO = nucleus supraopticus; NHP = nucleus hypothalamicus; NHD = nucleus hypothalamus dorsomedicalis; MMN = medial mammillary nucleus; NHR = nucleus hypothalamus retromedicalis; AC = anterior commissure; OC = optic chiasma; I = infundibulum.

Clinically this is evidenced by pain being elicited from mere touch. The theory explaining this concept is that repeated impulses from the nociceptor C fibers impinging on the dorsal horn (SG region of Rexed layers I and II) cause hypersensitivity of the wide-dynamic-range (WDR) neurons.[25]

The initial trauma causing the noxious reaction on the C-nociceptor fibers proceeds through the dorsal root ganglia and impinges on the dorsal column area Rexed layers I and II (SG). These bombard the adjacent area of the dorsal horn (termed WDR by Roberts).[25] The WDRs become hypersensitive, accepting impulses from the myelinated mechanoreceptors (Fig. 10–6), which now become nociceptive. Light touch now becomes painful.

There is also a neural connection within the cord where the WDR cells innervate the lateral horn cells of the autonomic nervous system. This circuit affecting the afferent autonomic fibers explains, in part, some if not all the dystrophic changes of RSD.

Because of these cord neuronal circuits, there are also synapses within the anterior horn cells that initiate muscle contraction ("spasm") at the segmental level. When excessive and sustained, this muscular contraction becomes an additional nociceptor. The vascular reaction of sustained muscular contraction becomes a sympathetic mediated nociceptor.

The cerebral mechanism of pain reception also involves the autonomic nervous system. Since the advent of *positron emission tomography* (PET), which localizes precise areas of cerebral blood flow, the precise brain region affected by peripheral stimulation[26] can be determined.

In PET studies, pain perception affects the anterior cingulate gyrus and the primary and secondary somatosensory cortices. Painful peripheral heat application[27] causes activation of the contralateral anterior cingulate somatosensory cortices. Nonnoxious stimulation activates only the primary somatosensory cortices. This would imply that secondary cortices are involved in pain perception, whereas primary cortices are involved in mechanoreception.

The anterior cingulate gyrus, which is a part of the limbic systems, is involved in pain perception including the emotions and affective responses.

In addition to the neurophysiologic aspects of pain, there is also evidence of hormonal involvement. This is termed *psychoneuroendocrinology*. The autonomic nervous system is obviously so involved, and the brain is actually considered to be an endocrine organ.

Neurotransmitters secrete substances, proteins or polypeptides, so similar to hormones that they have been termed *pareneurons*. Examples of these compounds include adrenocorticotropic hormone (ACTH), thyroxine, beta-endorphine, steroids, and so on. Acting in a tonic rather than a phasic manner, hormones exert their effects over a longer period of time than do neurotransmitters, which exert their neurotropic action in milliseconds.

Recent studies[28] have related *chronic fatigue syndrome* to sympathetic mediated pain. This theory pinpoints the following phases of the syndrome:

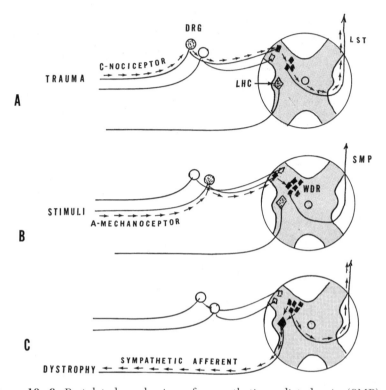

**Figure 10–6.** Postulated mechanism of sympathetic-mediated pain (SMP). (*A*) Transmission of impulses via C-nociceptive fibers from the periphery where tissues have been injured, releasing nociceptive chemical. These impulses pass through the dorsal root ganglion (DRG) to activate the Rexed layers of the gray matter. Impulses ascend cephalad to the thalamus via the lateral spinothalamic tracts (LST). The lateral horn cells (LHC) as yet remain dormant. (*B*) With persistent stimulus of the nociceptive fibers and the mechanoreceptor fibers, the wide-dynamic-range cells (WDR) become activated, sending impulses to the lateral horn cells (autonomic) and nociceptive impulses cephalad as sympathetic mediated pain (SMP). The hyperactive WDR cells now are also stimulated by mechanoreceptor impulses, causing the peripheral tissues to become hypersensitive (allodynia). (*C*) As the WDR cells become more sensitized, they stimulate the LHC, initiating afferent sympathetic impulses peripherally, creating vasomotor tissue changes of dystrophy.

1. An inciting event that stimulates the posterior thalamus, which is responsible for sympathetic action (fight or flight), occurs. These inciting events may (a) have a viral cause; (b) be brought on by an immune imbalance that is congenital or secondary to the viral invasion; (c) be caused by prolonged psychologic stress; or (d) be brought on by physical trauma.

These inciting factors, which are essentially nociceptors or algogens, initiate an "inflammatory" nociceptor process.[29] As stated in Chapter 1, they include lymphoid cells that liberate histamine, serotonin, bradykinin, arachidonic acid, and prostaglandin.[30] These inflamed nociceptors result in hyperalgesia[31] and myalgia.[32]

2. Progressive sympathetic flow results in a preponderance of sympathetic output. Whether the physiologic result of the output is organ-specific or generalized remains a question, but there is stimulation of the adrenals.

3. The sympathetic preponderance, considered an *up-regulation*, reaches the postganglionic presynaptic. Then the terminal autonomic nerves begin to "leak" norepinephrine from the vesicles that store catecholamines. This continued leaking decreases the sensitivity of the alpha-2 receptors. The balance between alpha and beta receptors is upset.

Patients with endogenous depression have an up-regulated alpha-2 regulation. It is here that the benefits of tricyclic antidepressants exert their effect. The value of tricyclic antidepressants in pain may also be in this domain as well as in the association of chronic pain to depression. Chronic pain and its relationship to chronic fatigue present another avenue of research.

The relationship of the autonomic nervous system to chronic pain has many ramifications that are not fully documented yet.

There is often aggravation of the local pain and referred pain from minor, unrelated, and reasonably innocuous stimuli, which are transmitted to the central nervous system via mechanoreceptors (see Fig. 10–6). These receptors and their afferent fibers normally do not transmit pain, but with sympathetic mediated pain, they enhance the pain.

The original trauma transmits action potentials through C-nociceptive fibers to the dorsal root ganglion (DRG), where they are then transmitted to the dorsal horn (Rexed layers) of the spinal cord. They bombard that region and form a hypersensitive set of neurons (WDRs). The WDR can then be bombarded by impulses from the mechanoreceptors from the skin, muscles, tendons, ligaments, and so on, which travel via A-mechano fibers of myelinated nerves. These later impulses impinge on the already hypersensitive cord regions (WDR), which can "spill" over, or influence, the proximal nerve cells (lateral horn) of the autonomic (sympathetic) nerves. This indicates how innocuous, unrelated touch pressure or movement can intensify the pain, even though the sensation is carried by mechanoreceptors, not nociceptors. These impulses then travel distally (efferent) to the periphery, causing vasomotor reactions as well as stimulating sympathetic pain sensations.

The vasomotor changes of the dystrophy that evolves are thus explained. Also explained is the basis of sympathetic afferent impulses initiating the cycle, which is then enhanced by mechanoreceptor irritants such as touch, stretch, and passive and active motion.

In the symptomatic lower extremity RSD lesions, which eventually develop a minor or major RSD, the etiologic concept may remain unanswered, but its occurrence demands attention, diagnostic and therapeutic, which is to minimize the disabling sequelae.

# REFLEX SYMPATHETIC DYSTROPHY IN
# LOWER EXTREMITY

Whereas major RSD causalgia occurs posttraumatically in lower extremity injuries, by definition, a partial nerve lesion must occur for there to be RSD and causalgia. In conditions such as fractures, dislocations, and poststroke hemiparetic lower extremity lesions, no nerve lesion is needed to have RSD develop. Regardless of the etiology, the minor RSD lesion of knee-ankle-foot syndrome usually does not have a partial nerve lesion or develop a painful causalgia. All of the sequelae of RSD can develop.

# LEG-ANKLE-FOOT RSD SYNDROME

In this condition, there is a dysfunction of the sympathetic nervous system, but from a different physiologic basis and from a different etiologic entitity. As a rule, this RSD is mechanical, stemming from a nerve pressure and a neurovascular response. The somatic nerve supply to the lower extremity (see Figs. 1–43 through 1–47) is accompanied by sympathetic nerves.

The normal circulation of the lower extremity can be simplistically divided into arterial and venous components, both of which have a mechanical component.

1. The arterial component is the cardiac pumping action, major arterial tone, and constriction-relaxation cycle, and the gravitational forces that propel the arterial blood flow to the distal portions of the upper extremity. The blood flow through the major arteries, and then arterioles, ends in the capillaries, where there is diffusion into the tissues.

2. The return of the circulation to the heart and lungs is through the venous and lymphatic channels by virtue of pump action. The muscles of the calf and anterior compartment literally pump the blood proximally with the assistance of gravity. Frequently, the leg must be held above heart level for gravity to be effective. The lower leg muscles thus act as a pump in this activity. The thigh, knee, and ankle muscles move the leg, ankle, and foot in every direction, as well as pumping the venous lymphatic blood elements toward the heart and elevating the upper extremity above the heart (see Fig. 1–49).

Repeated contraction and relaxing muscular action of the leg muscles pump the blood and lymphatic fluid proximally. Failure of either of these pumps to function adequately may lead to a painful and disabling condition termed *leg-foot-ankle syndrome*. Loss of ankle alternating flexion-extension eliminates the distal pump. As is well known, a fracture dislocation of the knee, with or without casting, may initiate this condition.

Pain from this syndrome varies and includes everything from an "ache," deep discomfort, tenderness, pain on movement, to even mild "burning." Pain usually does not occur initially or necessarily early in this entity, but it may only be noted several days to weeks after the onset. Most often, there are other impairments of function other than pain, which is why the condition is not diagnosed early in many cases.

## Mechanism of Leg-Ankle-Foot Syndrome

From whatever initial condition, the sequela of the leg-ankle-foot (LAF) syndrome is that the muscular pump does not function. The knee, ankle, and foot fail to move appropriately, and ultimately there is failure at an elevation above the heart level. Inadequate hip and knee motion impairs the upper pump action, and there is diminution of venous lymphatic flow.

There are many factors that may initiate limited motion:

1. Meniscus tears
2. Ligament tears: Collateral and cruciate
3. Fracture dislocation of the bones of, and adjacent to, the knee joint
4. Posthemiplegic knee-foot-ankle impairment
5. Postoperative casting
6. Soft-tissue surgical procedures

## Diagnosis of Leg-Ankle-Foot Syndrome

The knee and/or ankle may become "stiff" in that there is limited passive and active range of motion. The cause of this limitation must be discerned and addressed. Most of these causes have been discussed in this text and will not be repeated here. However, in addition to the many knee problems elicited, the following must also be considered:

1. Systemic paresis, such as that caused by Guillain-Barré syndrome, poliomyelitis, and so on
2. Spinal cord injury with paraplegia or quadriplegia
3. Inappropriate immobilization from casting or sustained position

The onset of the RSD LAF syndrome is first noted in the foot, where subtle edema appears on the dorsum and in the toes. The skin becomes shiny, smooth, and pale. At first, pitting may be elicited, but the degree of pitting is usually so minimal that it may escape attention.

Full ankle plantar flexion and dorsiflexion are decreased, as are the active and passive ranges of motion of the toes. Precise evaluation here also requires careful attention since the degree of limitation is so minimal that it must be compared to the opposite foot, ankle, and toes or its presence will escape attention. This limited range of motion is the subtle beginning of the loss of the distal pump.

Limitation of the toes and the ankle occurs from edema under the corresponding tendons.

At first edematous, the skin is also ischemic and becomes thickened and then ultimately atrophic. Clinically, there is hyperhydrosis (excessive sudomotor activity) early on. The foot is moist. It may either be pale or have slight turgor. The color changes depend on impaired vasomotor tone as to whether there is vasodilation or vasoconstriction. The foot is thus moist, pale, and cold or warm, and when compared with the other, normal, foot, the vasomotor-sudomotor abnormality is noted early in the condition.

Although the affected skin in RSD is more often cold (vasoconstricted) than warm (vasodilated), there is an increased blood flow in the subcutaneous tissues,[33] muscles,[34] and bones.[35] This increased bone blood flow may account for the increased activity noted in radioactive bone scans in RSD. This increased deeper blood flow also may initiate a transient arteriovenous shunt with decreased superficial blood flow, and hence the ultimate dystrophy.

The hair follicles also thicken (hypertrichosis) from excessive sudomotor activity, and the nails also thicken. All these sudomotor-vasomotor changes are, at first, subtle, but gradually progress. The stage at which they are discovered and treatment started determines the correctability or reversibility of the structural changes.

## Stages of Leg-Ankle-Foot Syndrome

Following is an outline that summarizes the stages of LAF syndrome.

1. Stage I: Vasomotor signs or hyperhydrosis with edema.
   a. Limited range of motion (with or without pain) in ankles and toes.
   b. Swelling of dorsum of foot and ankle: at first pitting.
   c. Skin becomes shiny: dry or moist.
   d. Limited range of motion of foot, ankle, and toe flexion.
   e. Pain on ankle dorsiflexion and plantar flexion.
2. Stage II: Most significant change in the edema is that it is "firmer" and cannot be dimpled by pressure.
   a. Foot and ankle pain may subside, and there may be a slight increase in the range of motion: active and passive.
   b. Edema of foot appears to subside but is less pitting.
   c. Skin is less elastic.
   d. Toes become stiffer.
   e. Nails and hair become coarser.

   **f.** Skin becomes less sensitive.
   **g.** Osteoporosis becomes evident on x-rays.
3. Stage III
   **a.** Progressive atrophy of bones, skin, and muscles.
   **b.** Limited passive range of motion at the ankle and toes.
   **c.** Nails are brittle and grooved; the hair follicles are large and brittle.
   **d.** Pain may now be minimal or absent except when passive motion is attempted.

X-rays that reveal bone atrophy (osteoporosis) may be noted early, even at stage I, but usually it is noted at stage II. Diagnostic x-rays should always include the opposite foot for comparison because early changes are subtle. Bone density studies have been developed that differentiate and grade the degree of osteoporosis. However, these are more academic because it must be stated that *the initial diagnosis must not be made on finding bone density changes in foot x-rays*. By then, stage III is in its early onset.

During the progression of LAF syndrome, ultimately there are atrophic articular changes. By virtue of the ischemia from vasomotor abnormality, the cartilage of the tarsal, metatarsal, and phalangeal bones impairs the circulation of the joints, and atrophic arthritis results. Furthermore, no motion, passive or active, is possible. There is no pain, but there is also no function of the ankle, foot, and toes.

Stages I and II are considered reversible to a practical, functional degree. With stage III, there are many irreversible structural changes that make functional recovery limited, if at all feasible.

Proper diagnosis requires inspecting the occurrence of subtle skin changes of the foot in any condition of the lower extremity where there is (1) an ankle "problem" of pain or limitation; (2) pain or limitation of the foot; (3) pain or limitation of the digits of the hand; (4) trauma to the lower extremity, such as surgery, injection, or a sprain-strain; or (5) a systemic condition with referred pain to the lower extremity.

## Treatment of RSD

Treatment of RSD varies only slightly when there is causalgic pain or not. Causalgic pain must obviously be addressed forcefully and energetically until overcome or significantly minimized. Without relief of causalgic pain, the syndrome cannot be remedied or moderated. Treatment of the sequelae of reflex dystrophy must also be addressed simultaneously and energetically as well as concurrently with the treatment of causalgic pain. To relieve the pain but retain a residual stage III foot would ill serve the patient.

Interruption of sympathetic hyperactivity is universally indicated. For RSD of the lower extremity, a chemical block of the sympathetic nervous system via caudal block has been considered diagnostic and therapeutic. Other forms of sympathetic intervention have subsequently been advised, but using chemical caudal block initially still prevails.

Sweet and White[36] suggested that, because of the prevalence of emotional factors in this condition, a placebo diagnostic test should be considered. After obtaining relief from a local anesthetic, but no response from sterile saline, then sympathetic interruption should be considered. Because the condition is so ominous and the stellate block (Fig. 10–7) relatively simple and safe, initial active treatment should be considered and undertaken. If severe emotional problems play a role, therapy in that direction becomes a significant part of the treatment program.

A series of epidural blocks should be considered. Usually a minimum of four is suggested, but more have been effective in specific cases before surgical extirpation of the sympathetic ganglia is considered. The decision to resort to surgery is based on the significant benefit to be derived from chemical sympathectomy and the patient's acceptance of the sequelae of a sympathectomy, such as ptosis and Horner's syndrome.[37–40]

Other forms of therapy may be considered and initiated. These include amitriptyline,[41] carbamazepine,[42] prazosin,[43] and local capsaicin.[44]

A provocative article[45] has recently proposed that a central control of peripheral inflammation exists. It postulates that two separate multisynaptic pathways subserve this mechanism, possibly being responsible for chronic pain in contradiction to the other concepts postulated.

This concept accepts that peripheral inflammation is initiated by local amino acids that act on non-NMDA glutamate receptors in the dorsal root ganglion. These activate both excitatory and inhibitory interneuronal circuits. The excitatory impulses are the ones stated as initiating the circuits to the hypothalamus, thalamus, and ultimately the cortex (see Fig. 10–2).

As these impulses increase, they stimulate more interneuronal circuits within the dorsal ganglion, including excitation of GABAergic interneurons, which are inhibitory in their function. If they are strong enough or maintained long enough, they initiate antidromic impulses back down the primary afferent fibers to the periphery. This is considered to be *dorsal root reflex*.

The amino acid nociceptors released at the periphery from this antidromic action increase the peripheral inflammation, initiating a vicious cycle. Within the dorsal root ganglion, other fibers previously "silent" become activated and also bombard the Rexed layers and simultaneously the peripheral receptors. The afferent fibers synapse on at least two neurons: excitatory (glutamatergic) and inhibitory (GABAergic) (Fig. 10–8). Though these events are reversible on interrupting any of the pathways, they may also present a new model for chronic pain.

Primary afferent fibers and sympathetic efferent fibers[46,47] are known to contribute to chronic pain. Activation of thinly myelinated (A alpha or type III) and unmyelinated (C-fiber and type IV) primary afferents can cause vasodila-

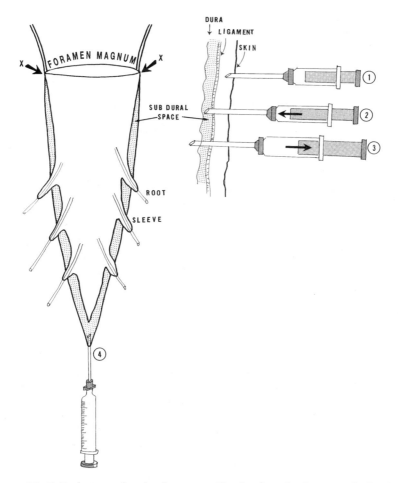

**Figure 10–7.** Technique of epidural injection. The dural sac that begins at the foramen magnum encloses the caudal nerve roots down through the intervertebral foramina. In performing an epidural injection, the needle penetrates the skin (1). As it advances into the epi(sub)dural space, the vacuum there pulls the plunger into the syringe (2). If the needle penetrates the dural space, the spinal fluid encountered is under pressure and forces the plunger from the syringe (3). The needle can be inserted posterially or caudally (4). Before injecting an analgesic agent, with or without steroid, it is important for the injection to be in the subdural (epidural) space.

tion and plasma protein extravasation.[48–50] If the unmyelinated C fibers are destroyed, plasma extravasation decreases.[51]

Neuropeptides found in A alpha and C fibers include substance P (SP) and calcitonin gene-related peptide (CGRP). These peptides have been shown to act centrally in the spinal cord dorsal horn but also to act peripherally, promoting plasma protein extravasation and vasodilation.

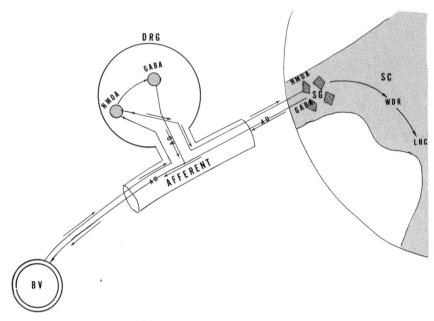

**Figure 10–8.** Excitatory-inhibitory antidromic pathways (schematic). Peripheral nociceptive chemicals released from trauma ascend the afferent fibers (C and A alpha) to the dorsal root ganglion (DRG). There they allegedly release NMDA (excitatory) impulses that act via interneuronal pathways to release GABA (inhibitory) that in turn activates antidromic impulses (AD) as well as excitatory impulses to the substantia gelatinosum (SG) of the spinal cord (SC). There, there is also a release of NMDA, which activates GABA and releases more central antidromic impulses. As these antidromic impulses reach the periphery, they act upon the blood vessels (BV), creating edema and inflammatory erythema as well as allodynia.

All of these factors explain the involvements implicated in RSD as well as in acute and chronic pain.

## VASCULAR CONDITIONS OF THE FOOT

### Diabetes

Podiatrists and other physicians are frequently confronted with complications of the diabetic foot. In the United States $200 million per year is spent on direct hospital admissions to treat diabetic foot infections with an average hospital stay of 22 days at a cost of $6600 per hospitalization.[52]

Diabetes is the number one medical cause of lower limb amputations.[53] Ninety percent of diabetic patients who undergo amputation also smoke.[53] The direct cost of amputation, including hospitalization, surgery, and anesthesia, is $8000 to $12,000 per patient.[54] In the United States, 20% of all diabetic patients who enter the hospital are admitted for foot problems.[55]

Diabetes affects 5% of the U.S. population, which is approximately 12 million people, of which 25% develop foot problems related to the disease. Diabetes with its complications is the third leading cause of death.[56]

People with diabetes who have undergone amputation have a 3-year survival rate in 50% of the cases.[54] With good comprehensive medical care and good podiatric care, the diabetic population could prevent ulcerations, neuropathy, and probably amputations.

Plantar ulcers and recurrences occur in 90% of patients who use normal footwear. Modified shoes and orthoses have decreased this complication to 19%.[55]

The causes of damage in the diabetic foot may be conveniently divided into three categories: ischemia, soft-tissue neuropathic changes, and neuropathic arthropathy. Vascular impairment, both large-vessel and small-vessel disease, with the former most prevalent, is considered the basis for diabetic foot problems. Because of arteriovenous shunting in the foot, the warm diabetic foot is considered to be at risk of ulceration,[55] and 40% of diabetic patients who present with gangrene have palpable pulses.[57] Of patients admitted for diabetically related ulcer infections, 80% have no systemic manifestations.

One-third of all diabetic patients develop distal neuropathy, and neuropathy causes over 40% of diabetic foot lesions[4] because sensory impairment impedes protective gait when a painful lesion has occurred. Diabetic neuropathy causes a loss or diminution of pain, proprioception, and touch. Impaired sensation, including loss of vibration sense, is a frequent impairment[58] and should be tested in all diabetic patients at frequent intervals.[59]

Complications of diabetes with foot involvement are ominous, as is apparent from the above statistics. When a diabetic patient says, "My feet are killing me," he or she may well be right.[7]

The preceding statistics are gleaned from patients who have amputation consultations and do not necessarily reflect the true picture of foot problems in diabetics.[60] The event of amputation is of major significance but does not in or of itself indicate the prevalance of diabetic foot problems.

Many diabetics have microangiopathy, which is responsible for diabetic retinopathy and nephropathy, but large-vessel disease is primarily responsible for ischemia in the foot of the diabetic. There may be claudication with rest pain relief, which suggests impending ischemia, but most commonly a painful, slow-healing ulcer is the most diagnostic. Faint or absent pedal pulses, dependent rubor, slow venous filling after limb elevation, and hair loss are also early diagnostic findings.

An ischemic ulcer begins as a small necrotic lesion that resembles a blister, usually found on a pressure site of the foot or toes. The center of the lesion becomes necrotic and sloughs, forming an ulcer with a surrounding erythema ring.

Ulcers (ischemic and neuropathic) have been graded.[61] Grade 0 has intact skin; grade I has a superficial ulcer that involves only skin and subcutaneous tissue; grade II ulcers extend to underlying tendons, bone, and joint capsules but with no underlying osteomyelitis or abscess; grade III is a deep ulcer with associated osteomyelitis, abscess, or pyarthrosis; grade IV has gangrene of the toes or distal forefoot; and grade V has midfoot and/or hindfoot gangrene. Radiographs are needed to determine the presence of osteomyelitis.

Various diagnostic procedures may be inadequate and therapeutic modalities ineffective.[62–65] Health professionals may not focus enough attention to preventive strategies.[66–68]

Simple preventive factors include the following:

1. Diabetic patients should always wear shoes when walking about the house.
2. Shoes should be properly fitted and maintained. Shoes should be prescribed after proper measurements of length and width.
3. Feet that deviate from "normal" should have specifically constructed molded shoes. All aspects of the foot need consideration.
4. Shoes should be worn with well-fitted stockings that are changed and washed daily with antiseptic soap. Cushioned socks are preferable.
5. Flat foam or customized insoles are desirable.
6. Frequent visits to a podiatrist or knowledgeable physician should be assured.
7. Education of the patients and/or spouse or parents must be initiated and repeated frequently.
8. Not all neuropathic ulcers are infected. Infection is suggested when there is local inflammation, crepitation, purulent drainage, and sinus formation. Fever, chills, and leukocytosis indicate significant infection.
9. On discovery of an infection in the region of the foot, specific bacterial studies must be initiated to detect the precise organism (gram-positive cocci) and discover anaerobic organisms (*Bacteroides*, *Peptostreptococcus*, and *Peptococcus*). Culturing must be considered.
10. Appropriate surgical debridement must be initiated when pathology is noted.
11. On detecting arterial deficiency, arterial reconstructive procedures must be entertained. Microcirculation abnormalities in diabetics have been questioned,[69–72] but macrovascular disease has been estimated to be present in approximately 16% of diabetics.[73–75] Arterial reconstructive procedures are currently used to augment wound healing and to obviate amputations, but this approach is not justified at this time and is pending further studies.
12. Osteomyelitis is prevalent in diabetes, yet plain radiographic studies are not sensitive or specific. Scintigraphic studies[76] have been diagnostic.

Studies are currently being implemented to systematically classify all of the factors that are involved in foot problems.[77,78] Potential causes and pathophysiologic mechanisms that play a role are neuropathy, ischemia, infection, and slow wound healing after trauma. Trauma, often minor, results in cutaneous injury with slow poor healing, ultimate ulceration, and possible infection.

The term *trauma* needs amplification since this can be subtle and unrecognized by the uninformed and uneducated patient. Current podiatric weight-bearing studies and gait analysis are valuable in detecting potential and actual trauma factors.[79-83] With these facts ascertained, special shoes and padded stockings[84] can now be constructed for more precise weight bearing.

Neuropathy and limited joint mobility have been found to be two main etiologic factors of the high foot pressures that are often found in diabetic patients with foot ulcerations.[85]

## Diabetic Neuropathy

Peripheral neuropathy is present in over 80% of diabetic patients. Because of the loss of protective sensation, ulcerations occur.[86] Because of the frequency of the affliction to the sensory nervous system, diabetes was originally postulated to be *caused by* the nervous system rather than the converse, which is now accepted.[87]

The precise mechanism of diabetic neuropathy has not yet fully ascertained. The early writings of Pryce[88] considered causes from retained toxic metabolites, vascular factors, and nutritional deficiencies. There are now[87] five pathologic processes considered pertinent:

1. Ischemia caused by atherosclerosis or diabetic microangiopathy.
2. Accumulation-inhibitory defect with lipid accumulation of fatty material in the Schwann cells that interferes with their activity.
3. Cofactor deficiency, enzymatic inhibition, or enzymic deficit, which affects the transportation of lipids and proteins.
4. Accumulation of sugar alcohols and glycogen, causing osmotic damage to the nerves.
5. Resultant thickening of the Schwann cell basal lamina and alteration of the nodes of Ranvier (Fig. 10–9).

Trauma affects this metabolic process (see Figs. 10–1 and 10–10). It is unlikely that there is a single cause for peripheral damage in diabetes, but from the above five factors, a working hypothesis may evolve.[87]

Impaired sensation, as well as pain and paresthesias, presents a major factor in the management of diabetically caused foot problems. All diabetics should be periodically tested for sensation. This can be tested by pressing a monofilament against the skin or by testing two-point discrimination (Fig. 10–11). If the

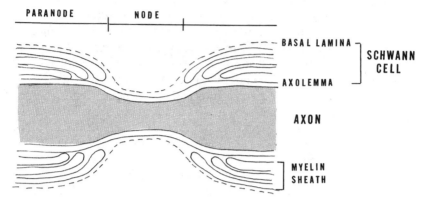

**Figure 10–9.** A node of Ranvier. The myelinated axon is narrowed at each node of Ranvier, formed by Schwann cells that invaginate to form a node, with the remaining portion being a paranode.

patient has lost this sensation, there is the possibility of ultimate ulceration. Loss of vibration sense is also noted early in diabetic neuropathy.

The most common mechanism of injury is the unperceived, excessive, and repetitive pressure on the bony plantar prominences such as the metatarsal heads (see "Metatarsalgia," Chap. 5), which are hypesthetic. Clawing of the toes also causes pressure-sore areas on their dorsum area. In the diabetic patient, any bony deformity predisposes to ulceration.

Neuropathic changes in the diabetic foot are a heterogeneous mixture of disorders including distal neuropathy, which is usually progressive; ischemic neuropathy; diabetic amyotrophy; and neuroarthropathy. The progression is a

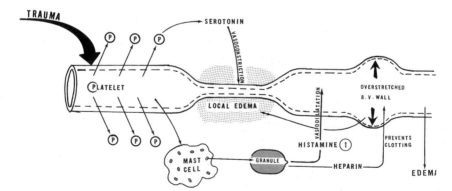

**Figure 10–10.** Schematic concept of vasochemical sequelae of trauma. The microhemorrhage or macrohemorrhage releases serotonin, which causes vasoconstriction and releases mast cells. The granules of these cells release histamine, which further causes vasodilatation with resultant edema.

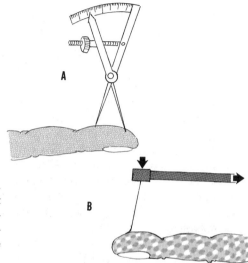

**Figure 10–11.** Light touch test. Using either (A) a caliper two-point test and/or (B) a Semmes-Weinstein monofilament discrimination test, sensation can be ascertained.

loss of light touch, vibration, pain, and temperature sensation. Initially, motor loss occurs in the intrinsic muscles, leading to claw toe exposing the dorsal joints and changing the weight-bearing forces of the foot. All must be monitored.

**Treatment of Diabetic Neuropathy.** The most satisfactory approach would be to prevent the development of the neuropathy because management of its sequelae is difficult. Adequate management of the diabetes with control of blood sugar level is the primary concern. Neuropathy appears to occur shortly after onset of the disease and subsides with adequate management.[87] If the patient can survive for several years with only moderate neuropathy, it is unlikely that the neuropathy will subsequently show any marked deterioration.

Avoidance of direct nerve pressure has been emphasized. The value of vitamin therapy, including vitamin $B_{12}$, remains obscure. Reduction of the body lipid content also remains unproved.

Neurologic motor paresis is detected clinically, and the resultant motor problems are thus addressed. This has been discussed elsewhere in the text (see Chap. 9).

## Management of Neuropathic Ulcers

Neuropathic ulcers are typically rimmed with callus and are painless. This latter fact causes many patients to delay seeking medical help.

Evaluation of a neuropathic ulcer must determine the presence and type of infection. If suspected, the presence of foreign bodies must be determined by palpation and radiologic and even magnetic resonance studies. Foreign bodies must always be suspected since sensation is usually defective and the initial puncture may not have been felt.

Loss of sweating and bounding pulses reflect the presence of autonomic neuropathy.[89] Evaluation of this vasomotor deficiency indicates the value of Doppler ultrasound testing.

Initially, treatment consists of paring away excess callus and topical application of 0.25% acetic acid wet-to-dry dressings. Avoiding direct and excessive pressure is important because this is a factor that prevents healing. Complete bed rest is unrealistic and actually undesirable because it diminishes the needed metabolic stimulation of exercise and the repeated elongation of collagen tissues in tendons and ligaments. Crutches and canes are partially effective. If the ulcer is small, foam inserts may suffice. A rigid sole diminishes the mechanical effects of toe extension on gait heel-off. An open toe box eliminates lateral and dorsal pressure on the toes. In the presence of a drop foot, an ankle-foot orthosis is valuable (Fig. 10–12).

Total contact casting is optimal if ambulation is to be permitted.[90–93] A slow and gradual transition from a cast to a shoe must be initiated with an interim shoe or sandal with a thick, pliant insole.

Debridement of a wound must be followed by application of sterile dressings. If the foot is casted, the dressing must be dry. A saline-moistened dressing of sterile gauze applied three times daily is recommended. Precise systemic antibiotics must be initiated and monitored. The application of topically applied antibiotics has not been conclusively proven to be effective.[94–96] Hydrogen peroxide, astringents, and iodine preparations applied locally have been found to interfere with wound healing.

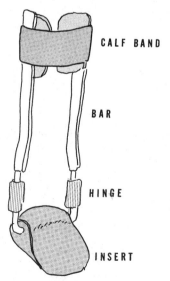

CALF BAND

BAR

HINGE

INSERT

**Figure 10–12.** Foot-ankle orthosis for drop foot. A short leg brace (orthosis) with two bars bent to properly fit the lower leg is held around the calf by a band. The orthosis is a fiberglass insert molded to the foot that fits into any shoe. In a diabetic individual, a properly fitted shoe is mandatory. The hinges at the ankle limit any significant plantar flexion or dorsiflexion.

Surgical correction of bony articular deformities of the toes may be needed. These include osteotomies, pins, and/or fusions. Amputations may be needed.[97–99] When there are toe problems, the midfoot and hindfoot must also be evaluated for their role in the mechanical deformity.

## Pain

Diabetics have a high incidence of mononeuropathies. Involvement of every nerve of the body has been reported. Many are entrapment syndromes resulting from local pressure, yet decompression, either motor or sensory, does not seem to benefit patients since many patients continue to have their pain after decompression.[100] Diabetics present a bewildering array of pain symptoms from local aching, throbbing, burning, to shooting pains. Pains appear to be most severe at rest and at night unrelated to any activity.

Diabetic amyotrophy is probably a neuropathy of spinal nerve roots that leads to motor weakness and atrophy as well as pain and hypersensitivity. Diabetic amyotrophy is usually encountered in diabetic subjects in middle or late life. It is manifested by asymmetric weakness and muscle wasting in the lower limbs, predominantly in the hips and quadriceps muscles, but ultimately affecting the lower aspect of the extremities. With appropriate medical control of the diabetes, recovery is expected.

Much of the pain in diabetic neuropathy is sympathetic in nature and must be addressed.[8] The most difficult management area of the diabetic patient is in the treatment of pain, and no one regimen has proved to be effective.[101] Anticonvulsants (phenytoin or carbamazepine) help some patients. Phenothiazine in combination with a tricyclic antidepressant is occasionally effective. In a localized nerve involvement, transcutaneous electrical nerve stimulation (TENS) treatment appears effective.[102]

More recently, attention to sodium channel–blocking agents (systemic or local) as being effective has been proposed.[103]

## REFERENCES

1. Bonica, JJ: Causalgia and other reflex sympathetic dystrophies. In Bonica, JJ, Liebeskind, JC, and Albe-Ferrard, D (eds): Research and Therapy, vol 3. Raven Press, New York, 1979, pp 141–166.
2. Paré, A: Les oeuvres d'Ambrose Paré. 2:115, 1840.
3. Mitchell, SW, Morehouse, GR, and Keen, WW: Gunshot Wounds and Other Injuries of Nerves. JB Lippincott, Philadelphia, 1864.
4. Letievant, E: Traite de Section Nerveuses. JB Bailliere et fils, Paris, 1873.
5. Sudeck, P: Uber die akute entzundlike knockenatrophie. Arch Clin Chir 62:147, 1900.
6. Leriche, R: De la causalgie envisagee comme une nevrite du sympathique et son traitment par la denudation et l'excision des plexus nerveux periarteriels. Presse Med 24:178, 1916.

7. Roberts, WJ: A hypothesis on the physiological basis for causalgia and related pains. Pain 23:297, 1986.

8. deTakata, G, and Miller, DS: Posttraumatic dystrophy of the extremities. Arch Surg 46:469, 1943.

9. Miller, DS, and deTakata, G: Post-traumatic dystrophy of the extremities (Sudeck's atrophy). Surg Gynecol Obstet 75:538, 1943.

10. Merskey, H: Classification of chronic pain: Description of chronic pain syndromes and definitions of pain terms. Pain 3 (suppl):285, 1986.

11. Tahmouth, AJ: Causalgia: Redefinition as a clinical pain syndrome. Pain 10:187, 1981.

12. Devor, M: Nerve pathophysiology and mechanism of pain in causalgia. J Autonom Nerv Sys 7:371, 1983.

13. Ochs, S: Axoplasmic transport: A basis for neural pathology. In Dyke, PJ, Thomas, PK, and Lambert, EH (eds): Peripheral Neuropathy. WB Saunders, Philadelphia, 1975, pp 213–230.

14. Perroncito, A: La rigenerazione delle fibre nervose. Boll Soc Med Chir Pavia 4:434, 1905.

15. Garfin, SR, et al: Compressive neuropathy of spinal nerve roots: A mechanical or biological problem? Spine 16:26, 1991.

16. Shawe, GDH: On the number of branches formed by regenerating nerve fibers. Br J Surg 42:474–488, 1955.

17. Wirth, FP, and Rutherford, RB: A civilian experience with causalgia. Arch Surg 100:633–638, 1970.

18. Doupe, J, et al: Post-traumatic pain and the causalgia syndrome. J Neurol Neurosurg Psychiatry 7:33–48, 1944.

19. Rizzi, R, Visentin, M, and Mazzetti, G: Reflex sympathetic dystrophy. In Benedetti, C, et al (eds): Advances in Pain Research and Therapy, vol 7. Raven Press, New York, 1984.

20. Ecker, A: Norepinephrine in reflex sympathetic dystrophy: An hypothesis. Clin J Pain 5:313, 1980.

21. Sawehenko, PE, and Swanson, LW: The organization of noradrenergic pathways from the brain stem to the paraventricular and supraoptic nuclei in the rat. Brain Res Rev 4:275–325, 1982.

22. Kalin, NH, and Dawson, G: Neuroendocrine dysfunction in depression: Hypothalamic-anterior pituitary systems. Trends Neurosci 9:261–266, 1986.

23. Ganong, W: The stress response: A dynamic overview. Hosp Pract 23(6):155–190, 1988.

24. Stokes, PE, and Sikes, CR: The hypothalamic-pituitary-adrenocortical axis in major depression. Endo Metabol Clin North Am 17:1–19, 1988.

25. Oachoa, JL, Torebjork, E, Marchettini, P, and Sivak, M: Mechanisms of neuropathic pain: Cumulative observations, new experiments and further speculations. In Fields, HL, et al (eds): Advances in Pain Research and Therapy, vol 9. Raven Press, New York, 1985, pp 431–450.

26. Talbot, JD, et al: Multiple representations of pain in the human cortex. Science 251: 1355–1358, 1991.

27. Devor, M: Nerve pathophysiological and mechanisms of pain in causalgia. J Autonom Nerv Sys 7:371, 1983.

28. Cheu, J, and Findley, T: Pathophysiology of the Chronic Fatigue Syndrome (CFS). Personal correspondence, UMDNJ Kessler Institute, 1990.

29. Rubin, E, and Farber, JL: The gastrointestinal tract. In Rubin, E, and Farber, JL (eds): Pathology. JB Lippincott, Philadelphia, 1988, pp 628–721.

30. Chahl, LA: Pain induced by inflammatory mediators In Beers, RF, and Bassett, EG (eds): Mechanisms of Pain and Analgesic Compounds. Raven Press, New York, 1979.

31. Pratt, RB, and Balter, K: Posttraumatic reflex sympathetic dystrophy: Mechanisms and medical management. J Occup Rehab 1(1):57–70, 1991.

32. Perl, ER: Pain and nociception. In Darian-Smith, I (ed): Handbook of Physiology, section I. The Nervous System, Vol III. The Sensory Processes. American Physiological Society, Bethesda, MD, 1984, pp 915–975.

33. Christensen, K, and Henricksen, O: The reflex sympathetic syndrome and experimental study of sympathetic reflex control of subcutaneous blood flow in the hand. Scand J Rheum 12:263, 1983.
34. Sylvest, J, et al: Reflex dystrophy: Resting blood flow and muscle temperature as diagnostic criteria. Scand J Rehab Med 9:25, 1977.
35. Ficat, T, et al: Trans M-A. Algodystrophies reflexes post-traumatique. Rev Chir Orthop 59:401, 1973.
36. White, JC, and Sweet, WH: Pain and the Neurosurgeon: A Forty Year Experience. Chas C. Thomas, Springfield, IL, 1969, p 87.
37. Fink, BR: History of local anesthesia. In Cousins, MJ, and Bridenbaugh, PO (eds): Neural Blockade. JB Lippincott, Philadelphia, 1980, pp 3–18.
38. Ladd, AL, et al: Reflex sympathetic imbalance: Response to epidural blockade. Am J Sports Med 17:660–667, 1989.
39. Dirksen, R, Rutgers, MJ, and Coolen, JMW: Cervical epidural steroids in reflex sympathetic dystrophy. Anaesthesiology 66:71–73, 1987.
40. Payne, R: Neuropathic pain syndromes with special reference to causalgia and reflex sympathetic dystrophy. Clin J Pain 2:59–73, 1986.
41. Max, MB, et al: Amitriptyline relieves diabetic neuropathy in patients with normal or depressed mood. Neurology 37:589–596, 1987.
42. Taylor, JC, Brauer, S, and Espir, MLE: Long-term treatment of trigeminal neuralgia with carbamazepine. Postgrad Med J 57:8–16, 1981.
43. Abram, SE, and Lightfoot, RW: Treatment of long-standing causalgia with prazosin. Reg Anaesth 6:79–81, 1981.
44. Simone, DA, and Ochoa, J: Early and late effects of prolonged topical capsaicin on cutaneous sensibility in neurogenic vasodilitation in humans. Pain 47:285–294, 1991.
45. Sluka, KA, Willis, WD, and Westlund, KN: The role of dorsal root reflexes in neurogenic inflammation. Pain Forum 4(3):141–149, 1995.
46. Lerner-Natoli M, et al: Chronic NO synthase inhibition fails to protect hippocampal neurons against NMDA toxicity. Neuroreport 3:1109–1112, 1992.
47. Levine, JD, Moskowitz, MA, and Basbaum, AL: The contribution of neurogenic inflammation in experimental arthritis. J Immunol 135:843s–847s, 1985.
48. Ferrell, WR, and Russell, JW: Extravasation in the knee induced by antidromic stimulation of articular C fiber afferents of the anaesthetized cat. J Physiol 379:407–416, 1986.
49. Kenins, P: Identification of the unmyelinated sensory nerves which evoke plasma extravasation in response to antidromic stimulation. Neurosci Lett 25:137–141, 1981.
50. Lewin, GR, Lisney, SJW, and Mendell, LM: Neonatal anti-NGF treatment reduces the A delta and C fiber evoked vasodilator responses in rat skin: Evidence that nociceptor afferents mediate antidromic dilatation. Eur J Neurosci 4:1213–1218, 1992.
51. Gamse, R, Holzer, P, and Lembeck, F: Decrease in substance P in primary afferent neurons and impairment of neurogenic plasma extravasation by capsaicin. Br J Pharmacol 68:207–213, 1980.
52. Wheat, LJ, et al: Diabetic foot infections, bacteriological analysis. Arch Int Med 146:1935, 1986.
53. Bohannon, N: Oral hypoglycemic agents. Audio Digest—Family Practice (audiotape) 35:26, 1987.
54. Bild, ED, et al: Lower extremity amputations in people with diabetes: Epidemiology and prevention. Diabetes Care 12:1, 1989.
55. Dyck, PJ, et al (eds): Diabetic Neuropathy. WB Saunders, Philadelphia, 1984.
56. Kosak, GP, et al: Management of Diabetic Foot Problems. WB Saunders, Philadelphia, 1984.
57. Nelson, RG, et al: Lower extremity amputations in NIDDM: 12 year follow-up study in Pima Indians. Diab Care 11:8, 1988.
58. Brand, PW: Ischemic foot ulcerations. Audio Digest—Orthopedics (audio tape) 10:7, 1987.
59. Gibbons, GW, and Bothe, A (eds): Diabetic Foot Management. Harvard Medical School, Cambridge, MA, 1988.

60. Sussman, KE, Reiber, G, and Albert, SF: The diabetic foot problem: A failed system of health care. Diabetes Res Clin Pract 17:1–8, 1992.
61. Wagner, FW, Jr: Amputations at the foot and ankle: Current status. Clin Orthop 122:62–69, 1977.
62. Boulton, AJM: The diabetic foot. Med Clin North Am 72:1513–1530, 1988.
63. Levin, ME, and O'Neil, FW: The Diabetic Foot. CV Mosby, St Louis, MO, 1988.
64. Brenner, MA: Management of the Diabetic Foot. Williams & Wilkins, Baltimore, MD, 1987.
65. Kozak, GP: Diabetic foot disease: A major problem. In Kozak, CP, et al (eds): Management of Diabetic Foot Problems. WB Saunders, Philadelphia, 1984, pp 1–8.
66. Cohen, SJ: Potential barriers to diabetic care. Diabetes Care 6:499–500, 1983.
67. Bailey, TS, Yu, HM, and Rayfield, E: Patterns of foot examination in a diabetic clinic. Am J Med 78:371–374, 1985.
68. Payne, TH, et al: Preventive care in diabetes mellitus: Current practice in urban health care system. Diabetes Care 12:745–747, 1989.
69. Walsh, CH, Soler, MG, and Fitzgerald, MG: Association of foot lesions with retinopathy in patients with newly diagnosed diabetes. Lancet 1:878–880, 1975.
70. Young, RJ: Identification of the subject "at risk" of foot ulcerations. In Connor, H, Boulton, AJM, and Ward, JD (eds): The Foot in Diabetes. John Wiley & Sons, Chichester, 1987, pp 1–10.
71. Tooke, JE: Blood flow abnormalities in the diabetic foot: Diagnostic aid or research tool? In Connor, H, Boulton, AJM, and Ward, JD (eds): The Foot in Diabetes. John Wiley & Sons, Chichester, 1987, pp 23–31.
72. Logerfo, FW, and Coffman, JD: Vascular and microvascular disease of the foot in diabetes. N Engl J Med 311:1615–1619, 1984.
73. Barlett, FF, Gibbons, GW, and Wheelock, FC, Jr: Aortic reconstruction for occlusive disease: Comparable results in diabetics. Arch Surg 121:1150–1153, 1986.
74. Janku, HU, Standl, E, and Mehnert, H: Peripheral vascular disease in diabetes mellitus and its relationship to cardiovascular risk factors: Screening with Doppler's ultrasound technique. Diabetes Care 3:207–212, 1980.
75. Wheelock, FC, Jr, and Gibbons, GW: Arterial reconstruction—femoral-popliteal-tibial. In Kozak, GP, Campbell, D, and Hoar, CS (eds): Management of Diabetic Foot Problems. WB Saunders, Philadelphia, 1984, pp 173–187.
76. Keenan, AM, Tindel, NL, and Alavi, A: Diagnosis of pedal osteomyelitis in diabetic patients using current scintigraphic techniques. Arch Intern Med 149:2262–2266, 1989.
77. Pecoraro, RE: Diabetic skin ulcer classification for clinical investigations. Clin Mat 8:257–262, 1991.
78. Pecoraro, RE, Reiber, GE, and Burgess, EM: Pathways to diabetic limb amputation: Basis for prevention. Diabetic Care 13:513–521, 1990.
79. Fernando, DJS, Connor, H, and Boulton, AJM: The diabetic foot—1990. Diabetic Med 8:82–85, 1991.
80. Fernando, DJS, et al: Limited joint mobility: Relationship to abnormal foot pressures and diabetic foot ulceration. Diabetic Care 14:8–11, 1991.
81. Duckwort, T, et al: Plantar-foot pressure measurements and the prevention of ulceration in the diabetic foot. J Bone Joint Surg 67B:79–85, 1985.
82. Boulton, AJM: The importance of abnormal foot pressures and gait in the causation of foot ulcers. In Connor, H, Boulton, AJM, and Ward, JD (eds): The Foot in Diabetes. John Wiley & Sons, Chichester, 1987, pp 11–21.
83. Apelqvist, J, et al: Prognostic value of systolic ankle and toe blood pressure levels in outcome of diabetic foot ulcer. Diabetic Care 12:373–378, 1989.
84. Veves, A, et al: Use of experimental padded hosiery to reduce abnormal foot pressures in diabetic neuropathy. Diabetic Care 12:653–655, 1989.
85. Veves, A, et al: The risk of foot ulceration in diabetic patients with high foot pressure: A prospective study. Diabetologia (Springer-Verlag) 35:660–663, 1992.

86. Caputo, GM, et al: Assessment and management of foot disease in patients with diabetes. N Engl J Med 331(13):854–860, 1994.

87. Thomas, PK, and Eliasson, SG: Diabetic neuropathy, Chap 47. In Dyck, PJ, Thomas, PK, and Lambert, EH (eds): Peripheral Neuropathy, Vol II. WB Saunders, Philadelphia, 1975, pp 956–981.

88. Pryce, TD: On diabetic neuritis, with clinical and pathological description of three cases of diabetic pseudo-tabes. Brain 16:416, 1993.

89. Archer, AG, Roberts, VC, and Watkins, PJ: Blood flow patterns in painful diabetic neuropathy. Diabetologia 27:563–567, 1984.

90. Cailliet, R: Pain: Mechanism and Management. FA Davis, Philadelphia, 1993.

91. Burden, AC, Jones, GR, and Blandford, RI: Use of the "Scotchcast boot" in treating diabetic foot ulcers. Br Med J 386:1555–1557, 1983.

92. Novick, A, et al: Effect of a walking splint and contact casts on plantar forces. J Prosthet Orthot 3:168–178, 1991.

93. Mueller, MJ et al: Total contact casting in treatment of diabetic plantar ulcers: Controlled clinical trial. Diabetes Care 12:384–388, 1989.

94. Steed, D, et al: Randomized prospective double-blind trial in healing chronic diabetic foot ulcers: CT-102 activated platelet supernatant, topical versus placebo. Diabetes Care 15:1598–1604, 1992.

95. McGrath, MH: Peptide growth factors and wound healing. Clin Plast Surg 17:421–432, 1990.

96. Knighton, DR, and Fiegel, VD: Growth factors and repair of diabetic wounds. In Levin, ME, O'Neil, LW, and Bowker, JH (eds): The Diabetic Foot, 5th ed. Mosby–Year Book, St Louis, MO, 1993, pp 247–257.

97. Harris, WR, and Silverstein, EA: Partial amputations of the foot: A follow-up study. Can J Surg 7:6–11, 1964.

98. Wagner, FW, Jr: Amputations at the foot and ankle: Current status. Clin Orthop 122:62–69, 1977.

99. Wagner, FW, Jr: The diabetic foot and amputations of the foot. In Mann, RA (ed): Surgery of the Foot, ed 5. CV Mosby, Chicago, 1986, pp 421–455.

100. Loeser, JD: Peripheral Nerve Disorders (Peripheral Neuropathies), Sec A, Chap 10. In Bonica, JJ (ed): The Management of Pain, ed 2, Vol 1. Lea & Febiger, Philadelphia, 1990.

101. Garland, H: Diabetic amyotrophy. Br Med J 2:1287, 1955.

102. Cailliet, R: Pain: Transcutaneous Electrical Nerve Stimulation. In Cailliet, R: Foot Pain: Mechanisms and Management. FA Davis, Philadelphia, 1993.

103. Tanelian, DL, and Victory, RA: Sodium channel–blocking agents. Pain Forum 4(2):75–80, 1995.

# CHAPTER 11

# Dermatologic Conditions of the Foot

There are numerous painful dermatologic conditions of the foot that interfere with normal foot mobility and gait. These conditions may be the result of mechanical compression and/or irritation. They may also be evidence of fungal or bacteriologic conditions, or they may be a manifestation of a systemic condition such as diabetes. Therefore, dermatologic conditions present a differential diagnostic challenge.

## CALLUSES

Calluses are a thickening of the skin as a reaction to persistent friction irritation with some compressive tendencies. Calluses are a dermal proliferation where the skin is adjacent to a bony prominence and little subcutaneous fat.

Abnormal foot mechanics are usually involved. In a "claw" toe, the excessive flexion of the interphalangeal joint and dorsal protrusion exposes the dorsum of the phalanges to the site of callus. In a hallux valgus, the enlarged head of the first metatarsal is also a site of callus. In metatarsalgia, where the heads of the second, third, and possibly the fourth metatarsal are prominent and not well padded, these heads are also a site of callus. A callus at the heel can be the result of ill-fitting shoes.

When a callus is confused with a wart, the differential diagnosis is done by paring and microscopically studying the tissue removed. In callus, the papillary lines that run through the hyperkeratotic skin are parallel and do not deviate and there are no blood vessels in the core.

In order to treat a callus, one must remove the offending pressure by either shoe modification, padding, or diverting pads. Pads over the callus have the center cut out. Diverting pads, such as used in metatarsalgia, have pads that cause pressure elsewhere than where the callus has formed. Periodic shaving of the callus may be necessary. Hot water soaks soften the callus, and direct application of a 40% salicylic acid plaster is effective.

# CORNS

Corns are nature's way of responding to the external pressure of the skin against the mechanical pressure from an adjacent bony prominence. They are similiar to callus. *Hard* corns develop on the dorsum of a toe from direct pressure there, and *soft* corns develop between the toes, where there is pressure but also moisture. The latter usually occurs between the fourth and fifth toes and in the web there.

The hard corn is treated by avoiding the pressure and by using the modalities advised for calluses. The soft corn is treated by inserting lamb's wool between the toes and by wearing a wide-forefoot shoe. Salicylic acid pads are effective. Surgical resection of the corn and/or of the bony prominence may be necessary.[1,2]

# NEUROVASCULAR CORNS

Neurovascular corns may pose a diagnostic problem. They also appear over a bony prominence and are sharply demarcated. When surgically pared, they reveal blood vessels "parallel" to the surface (Fig. 11–1), rather than vertical as in warts. They are usually very tender and painful. The neurovascular wart is best treated with surgical paring followed by weekly applications of 50% to 100% solution of silver nitrate. Between the nitrate applications, a salicylate plaster should also be applied.

# PLANTAR WARTS

Plantar warts differ from calluses and neurovascular warts because they are not found over bony prominences. They are sharply circumscribed with their edges clearly demarcated from the surrounding skin. Their center is darker than the surrounding skin and may have a mosaic appearance. The surrounding skin usually retracts from the core, presenting a visible cleft. Whereas warts, especially neurovascular warts, are tender, calluses and plantar warts are not tender.

Plantar warts do not develop hyperkeratosis from pressure. Instead, they are papillomas considered to be caused by a virus. There are different types of plantar warts.

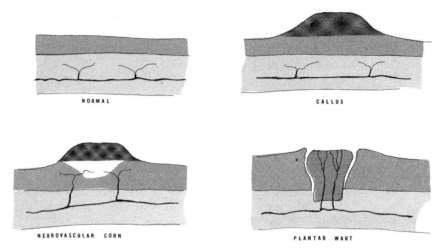

**Figure 11–1.** Dermatologic conditions of the foot. The *callus* is merely a hyperkeratotic area of the cutaneous level with no subcutaneous involvement or vascular involvement. The *neurovascular corn* is also a hyperkeratotic lesion with an avascular base near which are parallel blood vessels. The *plantar wart* is a papilloma, cone-shaped, with a cleft between it and the surrounding skin. The blood vessels in the wart are vertical, and the ends are visible when the wart is pared.

A *single* plantar wart that appears over a bony prominence may be diffi-cult to differentiate from a callus unless it is examined by biopsy. The margin then becomes apparent, and the surface is dotted by small capillary tips (see Fig. 11–1). A secondary *mother-daughter* type is a condition where a large wart is surronded by several small satellite warts. The satellite warts have the same appearance, but in their early stage, they are more vesicular than the mother wart. These plantar warts are exquisitely sensitive and painful. A third type, termed *mosaic*, has the appearance of a granular callus but is grouped in a mosaic pattern that extends over the entire metatarsal surface, unlike a cal-lus, which is over the prominence. Each mosaic core resembles a single wart.[3]

Treatment varies, but *surgery is contraindicated* for plantar warts because the resulting scar, which is predictable, is more painful than the wart and new warts grow along the incision scar. Applying salicylate tape directly over the wart and reapplying it on a daily basis usually relieves the sensitivity within days and causes the disappearance of the wart in several weeks. Or, the wart may be curetted and the exposed base cauterized with dry ice, carbon dioxide, or liquid nitrogen. Electrocautery at the base is also effective.

Mosaic warts are best treated by paring them down, at which time 100% silver nitrate is directly applied to the exposed capillary tips. This is followed by swabbing with a saturated solution of trichloroacetic acid. Following acute care, a 40% salicylic acid plaster is applied directly and maintained for a week. This treatment protocol is repeated weekly until normal skin is evident.

# BUNIONS

A bunion is a painful bursa that has become inflamed and its walls thickened from repeated pressure and friction. The underlying condition is addressed, and local measures are used in treating the inflamed bursa, such as hot soaks, pads, salicylic acid pads, and even surgical excision. Adequate broad-forefoot shoes are mandatory.

## TAYLOR'S BUNION

Taylor's bunion[4-6] is a deformity of the fifth metatarsal position, which produces an abnormal prominence of the fifth metatarsal head. The dorsal, lateral bunion results from shearing this prominence with the overlying shoe and the lateral-lying adjacent metatarsal head. The underlying podiatric problem must be addressed.

## KERATODERMA PLANTARIS

The skin of the entire heel sole may undergo diffuse thickening with painful fissures. This condition is termed *keratoderma plantaris*. The numerous etiologies for this condition range from atypical psoriasis to avascular skin in the aged to excessive barefoot walking on hot surfaces allowing a drying of the skin.

Treatment requires warm soaks followed by deep massage with a lanolin-based salve. If the cornified skin is excessively thick, it can be reduced by rubbing it with a pumice stone or an emory board. Deep fissures may be treated by the application of silver nitrate. Local antibiotics are ineffectual because there is essentially no absorption by the skin.

## ATHLETE'S FOOT

Athlete's foot is a fungal infection that spreads from person to person or by contact, for example, by a contaminated mat or towel. Moisture is needed for infection, which indicates why this fungus infection occurs between the toes in the webbing.

Treatment for athlete's foot is as follows[7-9]:

1. Keep the feet dry.
2. Avoid occlusive footwear, synthetic socks, rubber-soled shoes, or plastic insoles.
3. Use cotton or wool socks and change them daily or even more frequently if the foot is hyerhydrotic. Wash and thoroughly dry socks frequently.

4. Use shower clogs.
5. Use aerosol fungicidal spray or powders daily.
6. Alternate sneakers.
7. Disinfect shower room.

## SOFT-TISSUE TUMORS

Most soft-tissue tumors are ganglia formed within tendon sheaths.[10] Dupuytran's contracture, such as occurs in the palm, also occurs in the plantar fascia of the foot. Treatment is conservative until the ganglia are of such severity that surgical resection is needed. Ganglia are a mechanical impairment and not painful.

## REFERENCES

1. Fitzgibbons, TC: Foot problems in athletes, Chap. 71. In Mellion, MB (ed): Sports Medicine Secrets. Hanley & Belfus, Philadelphia, 1994.
2. Giannestras, NJ: Plantar keratosis: Treatment by metatarsal shortening. J Bone Joint Surg 48A:727, 1966.
3. Montgomery, RM: Dermatological care of the painful foot. J Am Geriatr Soc 12:1045, 1964.
4. Root, ML, Orien, WP, and Weed, JH: Normal and abnormal function of the foot. Clinical Biomechanics Corp., Los Angeles, 1977, pp 435–436.
5. Dickson, FD, and Diveley, RL: Functional Disorders of the Foot, ed 3. JP Lippincott, Philadelphia, 1953.
6. Du Vries, HL: Surgery of the Foot, ed 3. CV Mosby, St. Louis, MO, 1973.
7. Levandowski, R, Keogh, G, and Mullane, JP: Sports dermatology, Chap. 45. In Mellion, MB (ed): Sports Medicine Secrets. Hanley & Belfus, Philadelphia, 1994, pp 189–193.
8. Lillegard, WA: Dermatological problems in the athlete. Sports Med Rev. Kansas City MO, Acad Family Phys., 1993, p. 89.
9. Fitzpatrick, TB, et al: Color Atlas and Synopsis of Clinical Dermatology. McGraw-Hill, New York, 1990.
10. Cailliet, R: Soft Tissue Pain and Impairment, ed 3, Chaps. 10 and 13. FA Davis, Philadelphia, 1996.

# Index

A *t* indicates a table. An italic number indicates
    a figure.